SECRET SEX LIVES

SECRET SEX LIVES

A Year on the Fringes of
American Sexuality

Suzy Spencer

BERKLEY BOOKS, NEW YORK

BERKLEY BOOKS
Published by the Penguin Group
Penguin Group (USA) Inc.
375 Hudson Street, New York, New York 10014, USA
Penguin Group (Canada), 90 Eglinton Avenue East, Suite 700, Toronto, Ontario M4P 2Y3, Canada
(a division of Pearson Penguin Canada Inc.) • Penguin Books Ltd., 80 Strand, London WC2R 0RL,
England • Penguin Group Ireland, 25 St. Stephen's Green, Dublin 2, Ireland (a division of Penguin
Books Ltd.) • Penguin Group (Australia), 250 Camberwell Road, Camberwell, Victoria 3124, Australia
(a division of Pearson Australia Group Pty. Ltd.) • Penguin Books India Pvt. Ltd., 11 Community
Centre, Panchsheel Park, New Delhi—110 017, India • Penguin Group (NZ), 67 Apollo Drive,
Rosedale, Auckland 0632, New Zealand (a division of Pearson New Zealand Ltd.) • Penguin Books
(South Africa) (Pty.) Ltd., 24 Sturdee Avenue, Rosebank, Johannesburg 2196, South Africa

Penguin Books Ltd., Registered Offices: 80 Strand, London WC2R 0RL, England

This book is an original publication of The Berkley Publishing Group.

The publisher does not have any control over and does not assume any responsibiliy for author or
third-party websites or their content.

PUBLISHING HISTORY
Berkley trade paperback edition / October 2012

Library of Congress Cataloging-in-Publication Data

Spencer, Suzy.
Secret sex lives : a year on the fringes of American sexuality / Suzy Spencer.
p. cm.
ISBN 978-0-425-21936-2
1. Sex—United States—Case studies. 2. Sexual fantasies—United States—Case studies.
3. Sexual excitement—United States—Case studies. I. Title.
HQ18.U5S64 2012
306.70973—dc23
2012005724

PRINTED IN THE UNITED STATES OF AMERICA

10 9 8 7 6 5 4 3 2 1

Penguin is committed to publishing works of quality and integrity.
In that spirit, we are proud to offer this book to our readers;
however the story, the experiences and the words are the author's alone.

This book describes the real experiences of real people. The author has disguised the identities of
some, but none of these changes has affected the truthfulness and accuracy of her story.

To the lonely
You are not alone.

Chapter 1

· · · · ·

I've always hated touch.

I spent much of my childhood and youth screaming, "Don't touch me! Don't touch me!" as my uncle—by marriage, I feel I need to add—chased me around the dining table determined to touch me. My family watched and laughed, thinking this game of chase was cute and fun.

It wasn't to me.

Touch from women was equally horrible. My mother knew better than to hug me. But she was a typical mom who yearned for the feel of her child. So every once in a while she'd try to sneak a graze of a fingertip across my skin, and in less than a millisecond my body would jerk and I'd jump, never realizing what I was doing—or had done—until I'd find myself standing on the other side of the room.

I'm not saying that I don't like touch because I've been raped or abused; I don't know that I have or haven't been. I have no memories of such, even though I do know that I frequently behave like someone who has been abused. I had a gynecologist who suggested that might be due to the fact that I'd been around so many people who had been abused that I'd absorbed their feelings and actions. I once counted up how many of my friends had been raped or molested. I want to say the number was nine out of ten. But even with their histories of rape and abuse, none of them seemed to have this terror of touch that I did.

I asked my mother when this refusal to let people touch me started, thinking that if I knew when it began, I could determine the cause, and then I could deal with it. She just said, "You've always been like this."

So maybe I was born this way. I don't know.

But whatever the cause, and despite years of therapy with more than a half dozen shrinks, that's where I was in December of 2004, when I sat in my town house in Austin, Texas, and first clicked on Craigslist.org, the San Francisco–based website that connects people with jobs, apartments, platonic friends, long-term lovers, and seekers of one-night stands all over the world. I scrolled down its list of locations and lingered, then stopped, on Ohio, a state I hoped represented America in its deepest, truest red, white and blue. I clicked and stared at its personals sections—"strictly platonic," "women seeking women," "women seeking men."

I don't think I needed an entire hand to count the number of dates I'd had since I'd returned to my home state of Texas fifteen years before. I do know that I'd never considered meeting people over the Internet. After all, rapists and murderers stalk the net for victims. But I figured if I met someone over the Internet, and just talked to that person over the Internet, surely I'd be safe. No one would have to know who I truly was or where I lived. And there would definitely be no touching.

I scrolled down further—"men seeking women," "men seeking men."

Then, there it was, the personals section I wanted—"casual encounters." It was for those seekers of one-night stands, if not half-hour stands. Before entering casual encounters, I read the

Craigslist warnings that anonymous sex with multiple partners could increase one's chance of getting a sexually transmitted disease, including HIV, and that the casual encounters section included adult content. I swore that I was over eighteen years of age, moved my cursor to "enter," and paused.

* * * * *

Just a few months before I'd sat with most of my family at a big round table in my favorite Chinese restaurant. "I need a family meeting," I announced.

They turned and looked at me. We'd never had a family meeting in our lives. I took a deep breath. "I'm thinking about writing a book about sex." It was hard to even say the word "sex." It was a word that wasn't mentioned in our family, unless it was uttered in a tone of disgust.

They sat in silence. Each one of them was widowed or divorced and had been for years, if not decades. And I've never been married. I thought that was irrelevant, though. I'd be writing about other people's sex lives, not exposing my own—or the lack thereof.

My aunt, who was a church secretary, and my eldest cousin, who was a jail chaplain, emphatically stated that they were against the idea.

I looked to my mother. Her opinion was the one that really mattered. She'd been an independent businesswoman, and from the way she held her head, I knew she was running her internal calculator. She's always told me I'm the only one in the family who knows what she's thinking. When I read in her blue eyes that she'd hit "total," I knew her answer. She was for the book.

My youngest cousin, whom we'd always considered the least practical and thoughtful of any of us, sat quietly. Finally, he spoke. "You could use the book to teach kids." He was a teacher in a private Christian school. "Besides . . . ," he said, and he got very thoughtful again, "you're too old to be tempted by any of this."

• • • • •

I hit "enter."

I headlined my anonymous, one-paragraph Craigslist ad NEED TO TALK ABOUT SEX. I explained that I was writing a book about sex in America and looking for people who would be willing to talk to me, in detail, about their sex lives. I spent another five or ten minutes reading and rereading my ad, before finally hitting "send."

Now what?

I stared at my computer screen, then out the sliding glass doors and through the dark winter leaves of the live oak trees. I'd spent the better part of the last ten years writing "true crime" books about real-life murder, sitting with the grieving friends and family of homicide victims, listening to their stories, memories, regrets, loves, and rages as they talked about the ones who had passed on too soon.

I proclaimed that I wrote these books so that people could learn from what had happened—that denial of sexual, physical, emotional, drug, and alcohol abuse destroys lives and that mental illness is a real disease, not a weakness that can be healed by simply thinking positive thoughts. If we recognize these facts and deal with them rather than ignore them, we can prevent such tragedies from happening again. That's what I preached over and over again. But I was worn out from all the tragedy. I needed to laugh—and talking about sex made me laugh.

Of course, that was my cover. It's a lot safer to laugh about sex than have sex. At least it was for me.

At nine-thirty on a cold, rainy December morning in Ohio, thirty-nine-year-old Amanda walked into her favorite neighborhood breakfast joint having no idea what the man she was about to meet looked like. While she'd sent him a photograph of herself, in her newness to Craigslist "dating"—Amanda was recently divorced after fourteen years of marriage—she'd forgotten to ask for a pic-

ture in return. All Amanda knew was that the man was fifty-five years old and married—and had been married for thirty-five years. Most important, he'd responded to her looking FOR FUN & FROLIC casual encounters ad with the fact that he was sure her clitoris was located between her ears. Amanda translated that to mean that the way to an intelligent woman's body was to be erotic to her mind. That very thought was what had "won" Mr. M his face-to-face meeting with her.

A well-aged gentleman stood and walked over to her—though his walk was more of a swagger. He was tall, dark-haired, and had a mustache and goatee. Nondescript eyeglasses couldn't hide bold eyebrows and penetrating eyes. A button-down, oxford cloth shirt covered broad shoulders and a bit of a paunch. To complete his preppy look he wore khakis and a Rolex watch. Mr. M took Amanda's hand into his and shook it as he leaned in to kiss her on the cheek.

If he fucks anything like he greets me, I'm interested, she thought.

It didn't matter that Mr. M was obviously five years older than he'd claimed. She loved that he wasn't afraid to pull her close and that his hello was elegant, deliberate, slow.

They sat down and ordered coffee, both chuckling that they were too nervous to eat. "Boy, it's cold out today." Their conversation was mundane to start. "Did you find the place okay?"

But while the coffee still steamed, Mr. M asked Amanda about other men she'd been with and what she liked to do sexually.

"Every time you ask me a question," she batted her green eyes and spoke softly, "you have to answer the same question." She watched to see how he'd react.

He quietly answered a few questions, trying not to squirm.

Then, slowly and directly, she said, "So, are you thinking you're going to let me put my mouth on you yet?"

He paid for their coffee and they walked out the restaurant door.

While the Ohio winter wind and rain nipped at them in the parking lot, Amanda made it clear Mr. M wasn't going to her house unless he climbed into her Mercedes and rode with her.

"No, thanks."

But it was Amanda's rule. For some reason, she believed that a stranger who wanted sex with her would behave himself and be, as she put it, "a gentleman about my safety and security" if his car wasn't readily available.

Mr. M reached into his own vehicle before anxiously climbing into her leather passenger seat. He carried with him a bag full of shower gear and condoms. Fortuitously, Marvin Gaye's "Let's Get It On" played on her CD.

In Amanda's 4600-square-foot home, Mr. M stripped off his khakis and button-down shirt, and she immediately began performing oral sex on him.

For the next two hours, they had sex, twice, stopping only to rest and talk about what they wanted out of this potential arrangement. He wanted to meet for sex once or twice a month. Amanda was fine with that. And they laughed about their initial impressions of each other. She thought he was distinguished and funny. He thought she was cocky and overconfident.

After they met a second time later that month, he said, "Well, seems like this tiger is nothin' but a pussycat once she's tamed."

I clicked onto Craigslist to see if my ad had shown up. It had. I anxiously waited to discover whether strangers would tell me about the particulars of their sex lives. And it happened: a Yahoo! Messenger envelope popped up on my computer screen. I clicked open the message: "Please forward whatever information you've got to prove you're not a creep, weirdo, prison inmate posing as an author (those schemes happen all the time, ya know), and I'll be happy to talk. . . . Interested to see if you're for real or not."

It was from Amanda, answering my Craigslist ad.

My vow of anonymity lasted mere minutes. My name appeared

on my return email and Amanda recognized it. She wrote back, ready to confess as much as I wanted.

"I've been very, very adventurous, and don't know any woman my age who's had as many and as varied experiences as I have. Some golf, some collect antiques—I explore my own sexual boundaries as a 'hobby.' I would not characterize myself as a sex addict (and neither would my therapist—went to 3 months of counseling to see if we could make the marriage work), but I am someone who knows the joy of daily orgasm."

Daily orgasm? I went to sleep each night and woke each morning with autopsy reports and trial transcripts—the tools of my true crime writing trade—and a couple of stuffed animals—a teddy bear and a dog, to be specific—all of which comprise, I suppose, the bedmates of a single, workaholic woman/child. So I hesitantly, reluctantly, and embarrassingly confessed back to Amanda, "I'm shockingly ignorant about sex and have been celibate for way too many years. So think of me as this totally naïve person who you're having to teach about sex, which, in fact, is exactly what you're doing."

I'm not sure why I leaked that bit of my private self to Amanda, just like I'm not sure why I admitted that at nearly fifty years old, I slept with stuffed animals. Perhaps I admitted what I did because Amanda seemed kind and safe. And perhaps I admitted about my stuffed animals because that didn't seem safe. I want safety in my personal life and anything but safety in my professional life. Writing true crime had become safe; there was no longer any challenge to it. But sex, touch—that's not safe at all.

. . . . .

Amanda lived in what she called a "hypersexual world," though her appearance was deceivingly otherwise—five feet, three inches tall; shining, chin-length brown hair; a round, pretty face; and clothes like a banker's—professional, tailored, no hint of sexuality.

"Have you ever heard about/seen/been with someone/know someone who can do female ejaculation?" she emailed one of the sixty potential sex partners who answered her ad. "Some call it 'squirting,' but I think that's a pretty crude term. It's when a woman orgasms so intensely that a fluid (not urine, almost like male ejaculate, but more liquidy and much more of it, very sweet smell & flavor) comes out of her. It's not just a little bit—it requires towels. Well, when properly 'ridden,' I do that."

Amanda sought men who willingly explored non-ejaculatory orgasms and were educated in tantric sex. She described tantric sex to her Craigslist suitor as "very sensual, very erotic, very slow play, deliberate and teasing, almost savoring it to the point of agony kind of sex. Not lovemaking from the ooey gooey, Air Supply in the background, standpoint. More like the art of delaying the orgasm, building up and backing down repeatedly to save up and increase the intensity of it."

After coming off what she called a "weekend of extraordinary sex," she told me that tantric sex was comparable to going to church—"a spiritual renewal that connects us to our very cores"—and she saw it "as the celebration of the very thing that makes all of us feel our own skin around us in the most exquisite ways."

For women, Amanda explained, tantric sex revolves around the man withholding his ejaculation until he's pleasured the woman several times over. In its most fundamental practice, it *forbids* male ejaculation, calling it a waste of sexual energy that can prevent women from experiencing multiple orgasms.

But Amanda didn't mention the verboten aspect to her potential sex partner. She focused instead on the hopefully male-enticing idea that he could experience non-ejaculatory orgasms. "You don't 'blow your load,'" she emailed him, "but your body experiences the same sensation without the draining feeling that load-blowing causes. When done correctly, it's very possible for men to be 'multi-orgasmic' with the final one being the ejaculatory one. . . . From what I understand and have seen, it's sort of the crème de la crème of feeling connected to your dick like you've never experienced before."

Amanda had researched tantric sex—which has its roots in

3000 B.C. India, uses aspects of the *Kama Sutra*, and combines yoga, meditation, ritual, and intercourse—and female ejaculation on the Internet. She read books and watched videos about both subjects, after which she returned to the Internet to scrutinize the Web's personals and dating websites. Her goal was to "rediscover" her experiences with the boys she grew up with—boys she believed were playful, tender, respectful, open, and who practiced give-and-take in their sex play, traits she felt she hadn't experienced in the last ten years of her marriage. That marriage had included several threesomes, a fact she proudly promoted in her Craigslist ad.

Amanda had also consulted with her gynecologist and determined that she had a four-year window before it would be too late for her to get pregnant. (One of the reasons for her divorce was that she wanted children and her husband didn't.) She strategically planned to use those next four years feasting on what she called the "epicurean sex smorgasbord."

An Ohio State master's degree graduate and owner of a successful consulting firm, Amanda posted her first casual encounters ad on Craigslist two months after she and her husband separated.

"Please don't tell me about your stats—the size of your dick, your credentials for pussy licking, or the kind of car you drive," she wrote in her ad. "I really don't care at this point, and truly want to discover what I like about you on my own. My pussy's a bit small (sort of a glove-like fuck). . . ."

Within three days, she was corresponding with Dom, the married man to whom she'd explained tantric sex and squirting. Dom was a bit doubtful of her boasts of being a "wildcat." He believed she was a traditional woman who was set in her ways and reserved when it came to sex. Amanda forcefully corrected him:

"First, I was raised by very, very, VERY conservative Republican Catholic Midwestern salt-of-the-earth folk. I'm well-raised, well-mannered, well-educated, well-heeled, and well-bred. . . . So I can be a lady on cue, 'on stage' in a business setting, and always on the outside. I can speak in innuendo rather than overtly sexual 'cock talk,' because I think that's more tasteful, and because I've been schooled to read the cues of my partner before 'letting fly' with those types of phrases."

She informed him that she was a typical Gemini star sign with the dual personality of its twins. "I've always got another side to me that I show in very select, very private ways. I save the 'other side' for those whom I trust, or those with whom I share a common interest. . . . Because I was also raised with all boys and know the mind of a guy like some sort of spy from the other side, I become very open, very un-shy, and very adventurous in almost all ways sexually.

"If a man has the control and discipline to whisper highly erotic nothings into my ear during sexual play, I truly have a very difficult time even keeping a handle on myself at all—past partners and my ex could tell you multiple stories."

She bragged about a man who was still weak-kneed two hours after she performed fellatio on him.

"As to your theory about whose idea it was to try what with my husband (all 3-ways were him, me, and another woman), I did all of that to please him, true, but I was the one to initiate all of it as well. No, I'm not bi—I didn't have a fantasy about being with another woman. My fantasies were to really adventure with my husband in ways that were the 'dreams come true' sorts of ways for a guy. I did that because I loved him and wanted to please him."

Their foray into sexual exploration, which Amanda had hoped would bring them closer, sent them in opposite directions. "My ex really got into painted latex, whips, some bondage, and the 'bang you like a dirty fucking whore' sort of mentality." Amanda described such behavior as "very degrading, very hard-driving, macho asshole kind of stuff."

After typing more than five pages, she finally closed her rebuttal:

"I promise, I'm not some beatnik hippy chick who's going to need to dance around with a tambourine before getting into her birthday suit. Cock-sucking is Sex 101 for me. Am I good at it &

do I enjoy it? You bet—very, very much. I'm looking for someone with the strength of will & desire to do Erotic Arts 700—or wants to go there in very mutual ways. I'm very, very giving, very patient, and very open to being with someone who's at a more intermediate level. But, I'm looking to do the PhD thing in a major way."

Me? I don't dance—with or without a tambourine. But I was searching to do the "PhD thing" via interviews with my sex sources. Let me emphasize: via interviews *only*.

· · · · ·

Two days after Amanda and I met over the Internet, she emailed me an eight-and-a-half-page, single-spaced document outlining her sexual history. A half page covered her family background, education, and religious and political views. The remaining eight pages summarized her sexual "Memories & Milestones."

Amanda's first recollection of sexual activity involved a boy from her neighborhood. He was fourteen years old, she was a mere five or six, and he asked her if she "wanted to feel something neat." She replied yes. He lay down in the hay of her grandfather's barn and put Amanda's hand down his pants.

"I only remember thinking, *Wow—that really is neat. What's this part? What's that part? Why's this part so soft? Why's this part so rubbery?* . . . So we made a game out of it—sort of like 'I Spy,' but more like 'Find the . . . (whatever texture/part he described).'"

Uh-oh was all I could think, *another person who has been sexually abused.*

Despite the fact that what had happened to her was criminal sexual abuse, Amanda denied that she'd ever been molested. "I have had no trauma associated with my sexual development (other than getting caught in a couple of compromising situations in my earlier years before I got more savvy)."

Yeah, right, I sarcastically mumbled in my brain, knowing that sexual abuse victims often become promiscuous. If they don't become promiscuous, they often become celibate. I know those facts because I've studied sexual abuse probably as much as Amanda has studied tantric sex, thanks to my own curiosity about whether or not I've been abused, having friends who have been abused, and my true crime writing career. *Abuse and denial combine to destroy lives.* So I later pointed out to Amanda the fact that she *had* been molested and asked her about it again.

"No, I've never been abused sexually," she persisted, though she did admit that the adult Amanda knew that what the teenaged boy had done to her was a felony. She argued that it wasn't molestation because it was consensual, despite the fact that she'd been only five or six years old. "I was just as curious and into it as my uncle. I just didn't know it was 'wrong.'"

Uncle? At that, I realized Amanda hadn't been molested by a "boy from the neighborhood," as she'd first written, but by her uncle.

"That event sparked all kinds of exploration. . . ." She, her cousins, and playmates poked and probed one another with Playskool people "to find the hole that we were certain existed somewhere on our bodies."

In second grade, she and her friend Thomas, a fifth grader, entwined her Barbie and his G.I. Joe into sexual positions. "Eventually, Thomas and I began mutual petting and exploration with each other."

When Amanda reached fifth grade, she and a male cousin pretended he'd tied her to the bed and she was his sex slave. "I have NO IDEA where we got the idea, and there was only very light petting happening. It was more the thought, the fantasy of it that kept our attention."

Yeah, that and sexual abuse, I thought.

Amanda's parents were worried: "I could hear my father's drunken diatribe. 'That's just not normal. She's going to become a slut.'"

Her parents were high school sweethearts who'd married after Amanda's mother had finished college and her father had fulfilled his commitment to the army. Nine months and six weeks after their wedding, Amanda was born.

"Sex was NEVER discussed in our household, unless it was chosen as an 'academic' topic. Mom was a schoolteacher, so would talk about it ONLY when pressed, and then in her lecture tone."

Amanda learned more about menstruation from the neighborhood boys than she did from her own parents. What little awareness I had gotten about menstruation seemed to have been grasped out of the air mere weeks before my first period. Amanda spent her middle school years grilling her cousins and younger brother about sex and the male sex psyche. I had no one to grill and grilled no one, except in sixth grade when I asked my mother what the word "pregnant" meant. Only reluctantly—as if it were a dirty word—did she tell me. Amanda relied on her cousins and brother to safely navigate her way "OUT of trouble, but still INTO situations and scenarios to continue exploration"—petting outside of clothes, sometimes seeing "it," letting someone see her bare, fully developed breasts. I had no one to navigate me out or in. No one tried to kiss me until I was in high school.

I wouldn't admit *that* even to Amanda.

Chapter 2

. . . . .

Sean was a twenty-five-year-old nurse, who'd read my Ohio Craigs-list posting and knew I was researching a book only, not looking for a casual encounter. Still, he responded quickly. "Do you live in Ohio, too? Will you tell me about you, just out of curiosity? The same things you asked me . . . do you mind?"

I'd asked him his age, race, and education level; about his child-hood, parents, and siblings; where he grew up; how he was taught about sex; his sexual orientation; and his sexual history, including the first time he'd had sex, how his sex life had changed over the years, how the Internet had affected his sex life, his concerns over STDs and about religion—the informal list of questions I carried in my head.

"Do you need a picture or anything?" he said. "Or anything more personal regarding sex?"

I sat at my computer and thought for a moment, trying to figure out how to word my reply—how to say something without saying anything. I had no intention of telling this young man my sexual history, but I'd been taught in a college sociology class to reveal just enough about myself to make others comfortable in spilling their most personal information. I placed my fingers on my keyboard and typed, "There's really not much to tell about me. I'm obsessed with work and that's what I do most of the time. Otherwise, I'm with my family. I lead such a boring life that it's ridiculous.

"I'm a middle-aged brunette. I'm nothing that's going to make anyone's head spin as I walk by, but neither am I going to make anybody throw up. I'm really pretty invisible."

In response, he asked if I wanted to know what he liked about sex, intimacy, and fetishes.

"I feel so ridiculously nosy like I'm leading people to believe I'm trying to get 'my rocks off,'" I wrote, "but, yep, I need all this kind of info for the book."

I should have known what was about to happen, but I didn't see it coming. After Sean provided a very few basic facts—white, straight, "wonderful parents"—he asked me to tell him what I liked about sex and intimacy and what my fetishes are.

"I wish I knew what they are, Sean, but that side of me seems to have died. That might be why I'm kind of invisible. The good news is that it should make me very objective while writing this book."

Shit. I'd told him the truth. Maybe a case of the lonelies had blown in with the slight cold front that tapped at my office door. Then again, maybe I answered him honestly because I was trying to assuage guilt for—I don't know—being sexually ignorant? For not knowing what I liked about sex and intimacy? For not being sexually active in a world that seemed to think that *not* having sex was a sin? After all, a psychiatrist friend of mine had suggested I get back into therapy because I had no desire to get married or have any kind of relationship involving sex.

"Why did that side of you die?" Sean wanted to know. "Don't you think that that side is important to have, or important to find again if lost?"

I didn't want to tell him life, family, Texas, work, lack of self-confidence, the acne that mottled my face and made me want to hide from the world, the forty pounds I'd gained in my forties—ten pounds for every book I'd written. But even though I didn't want to tell him, once again I found myself doing it.

"I grew up in a very Southern Baptist family that doesn't approve of premarital sex. Despite the fact that I moved on to other cities, my family and I eventually ended up living in the same town.

"Their influence, my wanting to be approved of by them and not looked down upon or shamed—along with the lack of opportunity—combined to kill, or at least bury deeply, that side of me.

"Yes, I think it's important to have that side. God willing, someday it will be resurrected.

"But, hey, I'm the one who is supposed to be asking the questions here." And I asked him to tell me what he thought about premarital sex and what his hopes and dreams were when it came to sex and love.

Sean wasn't that easily dissuaded. "Are you married?" he wrote. "Do you think you could find that side again and if so, what would it take?" In fact, he continually asked me questions while dodging mine, which I'd read on various sex and dating websites was a proceed-with-caution signal. "Don't worry," he assured me, "I will answer all your questions. I promise, just give me some time. I just want to find out about you at the same time. . . . I do enjoy talking to you . . . send me a pic please, so I can see what you look like. Please?!"

·　·　·　·　·

I ignored Sean's request. I didn't want my sources to know what I looked like. It didn't feel safe. Besides, I was scared that if a young person saw—rather than just read—how much older I was than he, he'd cease communication. And I needed to know about the sex lives of all ages, young and old and in between.

The second night Sean and I communicated, he did answer a few questions, letting me know that he had an eight-inch-long penis of "very good girth"—a question I had *not* asked—and that he liked having porn at his fingertips via the Internet.

I asked him his thoughts on monogamy. "Is that a realistic thing to believe in these days?"

He complained that I wasn't answering his questions.

Oh, Lord, when pressed, I have a compulsion to answer people's questions. My mother—nicknamed "The Bull"—won't stop interrogating someone until her questions are answered. It's always been easier to spill all then resist her, because in the end, there is no resisting.

And my uncle took it as a personal affront if I didn't answer his questions. "You're a traitor to the family," he'd say whenever I didn't comply with his wishes, spoken or unspoken. Besides, he taught me that no one's going to do anything for you if you don't do something for them first. So I wrote back to Sean, "I'm twice your age. That right there just answered a bunch of questions for you."

"Is the Internet cheating?" he finally responded to my monogamy question. "Talking in chat rooms? Instant messaging? Looking at porn? I think monogamy is important in a marriage, yes. But does it always happen? Not always, no."

Sean argued that "many factors" might "lure a spouse away" even though that individual had never been a "cheater" before—things like what was going on at home, how issues were dealt with, if the mate cared for and was there for the spouse, and if the spouse was getting what he needed out of the relationship. For monogamy to work, Sean passionately insisted, there had to be quality communication, not just one talking while the other turned a deaf ear.

"It falls back mainly on the person who has the opportunity to do something that will ultimately hurt the other and what decisions they make," he said. "But it also depends on what is going on at that exact moment in time in that individual's head and maybe the 'other' person has been there a great deal more than their mate and [maybe] they never meant to hurt the other person because they love them but they just got confused and need another chance."

Suddenly, there was a twitch in my brain. I typed, "Are you involved with anyone now? Are y'all true blue and loyal together?"

Sean wanted to know if that involvement question was for the book or for me. By then, we were emailing each other so rapidly—trading numerous messages in less than a minute—that our communications were overlapping. He was just reading and responding to my email about my age.

"You're twice my age? What does that answer for me? . . . So how is my opinion on this subject of any matter since my opinion is not valued?" He raged that I was taking him for granted because of his youth. "As if being twice my age makes you out of my league or unavailable for me." He wasn't trying to be "rude or a dick," he said, but if I opened my mind and "closed off the feeling of what 'others' would think, then perhaps you would be able to find the part of you that you once lost."

I was taken aback. In fact, I was a bit frightened by his anger and defensiveness.

"Think about that," Sean demanded. "I'm just being honest, because it is much easier to bring out and find once you decide, hey, this is me and I don't care what others think. If they love me, then they are my true friends. If not, then I don't need them. Perhaps I am way off. You tell me."

I didn't tell him that he was wrong, dead wrong, when it came to my family. I didn't tell him that when you're single and childless, your family is the most important thing to you—at least mine is to me. I wrote back that my query over whether he was involved with anyone was for the book. "And regarding the twice my age thing, I wouldn't be sitting here emailing you if your opinion/thoughts weren't important. I just know I wouldn't want to date anyone twice my age. Sheesh, he'd be 100!!!" I also explained that I was "just trying to keep things on a professional level."

Sean apologized and admitted he was married, had been for seven months, and had already cheated on his wife.

Less than four hours later he emailed me, "i am horny. u can add that in ur book."

Since he said I could use it, I decided to delve into it more. I asked him to tell me about being horny, as well as about cheating.

His answer was "i am rock hard right now and need to cum more than anything and i have no release so i am suffering." But he refused to elaborate on cheating. It would take too long to type, he said. He wanted to know if he could call me to tell me.

"If you want, give me your number and I'll call you, but it won't be until next week," I answered.

Sean replied, "I would give you my number, but I can't get phone calls because of the wife, you know."

With that, my relationship with Sean ended, as quickly and abruptly as it had begun. That was okay with me, though, because I had Jim, a man who seemed nicer, less threatening.

．　．　．　．　．

Jim was a thirty-two-year-old married pilot who had responded to the same Craigslist ad as Sean. Unlike Sean, Jim quickly and directly answered my questions. He said he had his first sexual experience when he was eleven or twelve years old—masturbation. He constantly pulled down his pants and watched his penis become erect, "which it would do almost automatically." But once it became hard, Jim didn't know what to do with it . . . until he got a glass of water and a bar of soap to use as a lubricant. "The first time I climaxed," he wrote, "I wasn't sure what happened. (But I knew I liked it.)"

In fact, Jim liked it so much that he began masturbating three and four times a day. He still masturbates frequently, "but not like in those days." That's when Jim told me he's a private pilot whose trips usually last four days, during which he masturbates twice.

"When I'm home sometimes I will masturbate with my wife watching and that really turns me on. I have a thing about being watched. I think I'm a little bit on the exhibitionist side. . . . I fantasize all the time about being caught while masturbating. (Hope you don't have me locked up.)"

Though Jim admitted that it was a difficult fantasy to realize without getting arrested, "which is not a fantasy of mine," he had been caught a few times by hotel maids entering his room to clean. "It's sort of embarrassing and exciting to tell you this stuff (told you I was an exhibitionist)."

I don't think he was the only one who felt that way.

Until Sean stopped communicating with me, I was spending day and night juggling emails between these two men, often, literally, every one or two minutes. Sometimes I found all that juggling exciting. Not necessarily sexually exciting, but daringly fun—flirting-with-danger fun.

· · · · ·

Two days later, Jim sent me photographs of his pretty, blond wife and their beautiful, blond, blue-eyed baby son. In one picture, the entire family stood close together, dressed for church and the baby's christening. They were so clean-cut and good-looking—like the all-American quarterback, his cheerleader wife, and their perfect child—that they reminded me of the covers of the Sunday school books of my youth. In another picture, Jim, in khaki shorts and a white T-shirt, napped on the couch with his sleeping baby wrapped in his arms.

How dangerous could a man be who sent me sweet family photos?

Within the hour he told me his wife didn't like performing oral sex on him and he missed that.

"Is that why you're on Craigslist?"

"I'm not really sure why I check out Craigslist occasionally," he said. "I guess I entertain the idea of being with someone else—purely for sex—yet I'm probably too chicken to actually do anything, so I guess I sort of flirt with the idea."

Jim and his wife had been together for six years—three years of marriage and three years before that. He claimed he'd never cheated on her, but since she'd had the baby . . .

"The problem is I'm as horny as ever and still want it all the time. . . . I'm yearning for some sexual excitement but can't get any satisfaction without breaking my wedding vows. It's frustrating."

Twelve minutes later, the married pilot asked me for a photograph.

I must admit, I was grinning a bit as I sat at my computer. Despite the fact that I had no idea if what Jim and Sean were telling me bore any resemblance to the truth, it felt good to have their (perhaps) sexual attention. It'd been so long. . . .

Chapter 3

· · · · ·

"1. Fully Surrendered Pussy-Licking," Amanda typed after her second sexual encounter with the married Mr. M. She was emailing him what she called her "drip list"—things that made her drip sexually. "Love it if I can get there."

I read her words with laughter and a wisp of envy—envy in knowing that she'd probably get what she wanted.

"I certainly have in the past . . . ," she said.

In truth, what I really envied was her sexual self-confidence.

But I have also been with some men where I just never could get to that fully surrendered point (hubby was one, unfortunately). I think it has something do with the enjoyment factor. . . . If I feel like someone wants to do it as a power play, or out of a sense of obligation, I'd rather just skip it and move on to something else. If someone truly enjoys it, and WANTS to do it, I surrender much more willingly.

2. OUTSIDE

There's NO FEELING like spreading my legs and having the sunshine & fresh air touch my readied body.

3. SEMI-PUBLIC SEX

A sex club seems to make the most sense (as to where to have that), from what I am aware of at this point. I want to go to the one in Dayton very, very much. I'm turned on by the idea of having sex somewhere that someone can watch if they want to. But, I'd prefer for it to be strangers—not someone I know. If it'd be strangers, I know myself enough to know that I'd relax more and get into my partner while ignoring those around me. If someone I knew would watch, I'd be too uptight about them "respecting me in the morning" (for lack of a better way to describe it).

4. FINE DINING + NAUGHTY TALK

Love fine dining. Love naughty talk. Would love to combine the two and see what happens. Would it lead to public sex? Don't know, but willing to see.

5. ARTSY SEX

I have no idea why, but anytime I'm in the presence of art, it's all I can do not to touch myself or someone else. . . .

6. HIGHWAY SEX

I have a fantasy to pull off to the side of a highway (like I-71—I mean a MAJOR interstate) in the "emergency only" lane, and go at it.

7. BLUESY SEX

Blues music also makes me hot in indescribable ways (New Orleans is my favorite city—but, Chicago's a close second). I once saw a band that had a saxophone player that was so good I almost had to go masturbate in the ladies room. I was with hubby at the time, so I leaned over to him, didn't say a word, but sucked his earlobe for a loooonnng time. He didn't get the hint (never did), but I would've fucked him in the parking garage before he ever even got the key in the ignition.

8. GOURMET SEX

This doesn't really have any specific setting or acts in particular. It's just the desire to have really, really good, mutually satisfying and trusting yet uninhibited sex. Sort of like when a good cook can't tell you a recipe, but creates dishes that make your taste buds sing. I have a friend who cooks like that, and it's sometimes difficult not to get turned on when he's doing his thing in the kitchen. . . .

What are some things on your list? I'm dying to know.

Okay, second truth: I envied her comfort with sex . . . her ease with getting turned on . . . and the fact that she *could* drip, because I couldn't imagine dripping . . . or having a drip list. But my own imagination wasn't the subject. Other people's sex lives was. So when Jim emailed me and wanted to know what other "dirty secrets" I wanted from him, I merrily went back to work and asked if he'd ever tried partner-swapping.

"No," he said. "The wife would never go for it." He wasn't sure he would either. "But I would love to bring another woman into the bedroom (every guy's fantasy)."

I tried not to smile as I wondered if he was hinting at something about me. Just because one doesn't like touch doesn't mean one doesn't want to be found desirable. Admittedly, I'd been tempted to send him a photograph. But I'd resisted the urge knowing it would be wiser to act with my brain rather than an aging ego. "Have you ever been with two women at once?" I asked.

Jim hadn't, but he "suspected" his wife might go for it "after a few beers." During sex she would sometimes say she wanted to "eat another woman's pussy." He wasn't sure she said that because she meant it or because she knew it turned him on. "Big difference from saying something and actually doing it."

He then offered to let me interview him "face-to-face" if he ever flew to my city.

"That'd be great," I typed. "Austin," I revealed to this man I'd "known" for all of three days. Yet I pictured us huddled together at a small corner table in the dimness of a smoky hotel bar. I wasn't sure whether my tape recorder was there as we talked. My mind's-eye picture got as murky as the smoke when it came to closing time. Did I go with him up to his room? I know I thought he was cute.

And I know I'd sat across from my shrink—yes, as my psychiatrist friend had suggested I do, I was back in therapy, going once a week—and laughed, "Maybe I'll find someone to date while working on this book." After all, dating, sex and relationships were the primary reasons I sat in my psychiatrist's office, again, as per the advice from my shrink friend . . . and despite my youngest cousin's comment that I was too old to be tempted by such.

Instead of going along with my jesting when I'd said, "Maybe I'll find someone to date while working on this book," my shrink had had a conniption.

"You can't do that," she'd commanded, her voice hard, her words clipped.

I couldn't see why not . . . as long as I didn't include that person in the book. After all, through work was the only way I ever met anyone. Maybe in researching something other than murder, I'd meet someone other than criminals and criminal attorneys. Maybe I'd meet someone normal.

Lord, what was I thinking?

Besides, as Jim said, there's a big difference between saying something and doing it.

· · · · ·

"Last night . . . ," Jim wrote, "I whispered in [my wife's] ear that I had been fantasizing about another woman going down on her, and we both came together. . . . I know it turns her on to think about it. But would she ever actually let another woman into our bedroom? And how do I initiate it and make her feel comfortable at the same time?"

I didn't know what to say to Jim. Or perhaps I didn't know what I *should* say. I wasn't at my professional journalist best that day. Hell, I wasn't at any sort of best, because I received that email on the actual day of my fiftieth birthday. *50.* The big, dreaded, AARP-membership-inducting Five-O.

· · · · ·

I don't recall a thing about that birthday. It's not that I was drunk. It's just that it wasn't worth remembering. There's not even anything written in my calendar that day. I have only Jim's email. If I had to guess, I'd guess I spent the evening with my family eating steak, drinking Diet Coke, then having grocery store white cake with butter cream frosting and washing it down with two-percent milk.

Several days after my birthday, I finally wrote Jim again. "How's it going now? Have you figured out if/how you're going to approach your wife about this?"

"I don't know how people can make that move," he replied. "And even if she was interested, how would I find someone?"

Despite the fact that I could grow a bit giddy believing that this young, handsome pilot was making sexual overtures to this fifty-year-old, I buttoned myself up and typed, "Jim, if I tried to answer that question for you, I'd be crossing professional boundaries. It's kosher for me to listen only. But feel free to think it through and 'out loud' with me. I do hear your frustration and longing. Does your wife? Have you expressed to her what you've expressed to me?"

Jim later admitted that he and his wife hadn't talked in a long time about including another woman and remarked that their sex life "used to be a little more adventurous. We used to even have anal sex. She used to ask me for that. And she used to have unbelievable orgasms when we did that."

But that was all before their son was born.

"Now [our sex life is] much more tame. Even this morning I asked her if she masturbated while I was gone on my trip and she acted annoyed at me for even asking the question."

That night, however, after Jim and I logged off from each other, he suggested to his wife that they watch a pornographic video together.

"We watched for maybe 20 minutes just sort of massaging one another." She masturbated, and he rubbed inside her until she had an orgasm. Then he climbed on top of her. "And we started fucking. She was so wet and it felt great." She rolled on top of him and "rode" him "really well." As he got closer and closer to coming, he asked her to tell him she fantasizes about women. She told him. He asked her to tell him she wanted another girl to "eat her out!" She sort of smiled and said she couldn't say that. He moaned, "Please." She said it, and he immediately orgasmed.

• • • • •

Jim later emailed me, "As you already know I am an exhibitionist and it gives me a charge to tell you my intimate experiences. (I end up getting a very hard erection every time I email you.) And you do enter my thoughts when I masturbate. . . . I did see a picture of you on the web and I think you are attractive. I hope I'm not embarrassing you. Just thought I would tell you everything."

Twelve minutes later I typed him, "Well, I do have to admit that the ego-stroking, no pun intended, is kind of nice, especially considering the birthday I just celebrated." I told him not to pay too much attention to those Internet photos—they were probably five years and thirty pounds ago. "I'm definitely no competition for your wife."

The next day, my shrink scolded me. I was encouraging Jim with my flirtation, she said. I didn't see it that way—as flirtation. I felt more like a starving old dog snapping up a fallen bread crumb and saying thank you for the crust.

Still, she was my shrink and I was paying her big buckaroos for her help. So I heeded her words and approached my psychiatrist friend for more detailed—and free—suggestions as to how to deal with my sources, whom my friend referred to as "sexually 'out there' people."

"You need to be careful about having any sort of relationship with them at all," she said. "Like the masturbator—you said it was flattering or something to that effect. He will take that as a green light to get more sexually seductive with you. Tread carefully with these people. They usually have very poor boundaries."

But I knew I was the one who had poor boundaries—in life, in relationships, and in sex. More than once I'd found myself in an unexpected sexual situation and been frozen in confusion. The first time I recall was as a teenager. I was at home, alone, lying on the couch, watching TV. Through the windows of our den, I saw a young man working on our house. Through the windows, he saw me lying on the couch in my T-shirt and cut-off jeans. He walked inside and, wordlessly, over to me, where he stopped and stood, inches away. I looked up. His skin was smooth across a handsome face. His wedding band shined silver against tanned fingers. He reached down and touched the tips of those fingers along the length of my bare legs. Hesitantly, he stopped and pulled back, but he still looked at me.

I didn't say a thing. Strangely enough, part of me wanted him to touch me, but I knew it was wrong. It was wrong because he was married. It was wrong because he was so much older than I. It was wrong because I was too young for this. But it was also confusing, and interesting, and enticing, and curious because he wanted to touch me; I wasn't the type of girl that guys expressed interest in touching. But the real reason I let him slide his tanned hand softly up my leg was that I didn't know what to say to stop him. And I certainly didn't know a polite way to stop him so that I didn't make him angry.

Thank God, he stopped himself and walked out the door, never saying a word.

· · · · ·

Later that week Jim mentioned he'd gone online searching for women who'd be interested in a threesome. He'd included, he said, pictures of himself and his wife. "One very beautiful 33-year-old girl responded. She wanted to see pics of me naked so I took some pics of myself and sent them to her. She said she liked what she saw, thank god, and that she was more interested in [my wife]. I don't blame her."

He claimed that he'd asked the woman for advice regarding how to broach the threesome subject with his wife. "She wasn't very helpful. Anyways, I guess I hit another dead end. Do you want to see the pics?"

I didn't respond to his question. Instead, I shared his email with my two most-trusted friends—my shrink friend and a bisexual friend. I'll call them Lola and Rose.

"Do you want to see his pics?" Rose asked me. "Tell him you're not an advice columnist. You are GATHERING information, not dispensing it."

I didn't answer her question either. I didn't want to admit that just like with the married workman decades before, I was curious. Part of me sort of did want to see the photographs, but I also knew that I shouldn't want to see them, and because of that I didn't want to see them. But then again . . .

Lola told me to say "No, thank you, I don't need the pictures, but I'd love to hear how the subject progresses with your wife." That phrase, "I don't need the pictures," she said, ignored "the fact that he's implying you might just want to see them because you want to see his huge one." Ignoring, she believed, was a good thing.

I heeded part of her counsel. I didn't answer his question. But neither did I say I didn't need the pictures. I asked him where he'd found his threesome advisor. I wasn't so sure he hadn't made her up.

Two days later Jim sent me five photographs with the note, "Don't laugh too hard."

In the first picture, he lazily lay in his black iron bed, thick white comforters around him, and stared dreamy-eyed into the camera, naked, while he held his erect penis in his right hand as though he were masturbating. The second picture focused on his testicles and scrotum, while the third looked like he was about to come. The last two were close-ups of his penis emphasizing its length and girth.

· · · · ·

When I was a teenager in the 1970s, I walked into a darkly lit head shop in Eugene, Oregon. The odd pungency of East Indian incense filled the room. Free-flowing clothes made of Indian batik hung on the racks. And I tried to casually study the black light posters depicting sexual intercourse positions derived from the *Kama Sutra*.

To me, the *Kama Sutra* and drawings of intercourse seemed wild. I was a high school student, in Eugene on a summer mission trip with my church. So when I walked into that head shop, I certainly couldn't stand, stare, and study a poster of sexual positions. Now, more than thirty years later, Jim's erect penis stared at me over my computer screen. And just like when I was a teenager, part of me wanted to race away and part of me wanted to study him out of the corners of my eyes.

I dutifully emailed him back: "Hey, Jim, I don't need sex photos. Words for my book are all I need. Suzy."

I told my shrink about Jim's pictures. Shaming words exploded out of her mouth. Sending me lewd unsolicited photos was the equivalent of Internet rape, I understood her to say. Worse, it was my fault because I'd flirted back with him and hadn't replied to his email asking if I wanted to see the pictures—I should have replied rapidly and specifically, stating an absolute no, don't send me your naked pictures.

By then, it didn't really matter. Jim had quit emailing me after

I'd told him I needed words only. But sometimes at night, I pulled up his photographs on my computer and stared at them. His skin was pale. His young body was fit. His thighs were long and firm, and I could almost feel myself wanting to slide my fingers down them. And his penis . . . all I can say is oh, my. It was beautiful perfection.

Chapter 4

· · · · ·

At nine-thirty on a January night in San Diego, California, forty-one-year-old Richard knocked on the door of a Marriott hotel room. He was far from completely comfortable with the sex he was about to have. But he was even more apprehensive about the people he was about to meet. Are they legit? Are they going to steal my wallet while I'm not looking? Is she attractive?

Earlier in the week, Richard had sat at his computer cruising Craigslist casual encounters when a posting caught his interest— NSA 3RD NEEDED-MW4M-35. *Translated, it meant a thirty-five-year-old man and a thirty-five-year-old woman were looking for a man to have no-strings-attached sex with them. Richard responded and attached photos of himself—including several pictures of his penis. The wife nixed him as a potential partner because his organ was too large.*

But on Friday afternoon, he received another email from the wife asking if he was available that very night. Richard was, and that started a quick exchange of messages.

"My husband will be involved also!" she wrote.

"He doesn't want to get involved with me, does he?" Richard

replied. Then he offered to send her additional pictures of himself to ensure she'd be attracted to him. He was concerned that would be a problem, even though he had no idea if he'd be attracted to her. She'd refused to provide him with any photos, saying they'd previously had a bad experience with such.

She, however, accepted his photo offer.

The door swung open and there stood Tabitha, the wife, a rum and Coke in her hand, her brown hair hanging long and curly. She was pretty, Richard thought—not gorgeous, but pretty. She was five feet, two inches tall and 127 pounds. She wore a light blue baby doll negligee that exposed her buttocks when she leaned over to freshen her drink.

Tabitha's husband, Bob, a tattooed, six-foot tall, two-hundred-pound man with a mustache, goatee, and well-styled hair, sat sipping a margarita.

Richard—tall, slim, firm, and nice-looking—mixed himself a drink and edged over to the foot of the bed. He already knew the rules for the evening. Tabitha had outlined them in an email: there would be no kissing because it was too personal, no anal sex, no pain, nothing involving bodily wastes, and no ejaculating into her mouth. Anything else, she was open to. But she had wanted to know if Richard would allow Bob to videotape Richard having sex with her.

Richard would as long as they had a mask to hide his identity. Tabitha had said they didn't have a mask.

For the next twenty minutes, Richard, Tabitha, and Bob sipped their cocktails and talked. Bob was a civilian contractor for the navy. Tabitha was divorced. Her son was a soccer star and her eighteen-year-old daughter was home babysitting Tabitha and Bob's twelve-month-old baby.

Once before, in fact, just the week before, Tabitha and her husband had tried a threesome. But it hadn't worked out—the invited man hadn't been able to "perform."

Tabitha rose out of her chair, walked over to Richard, and

unzipped his pants. Richard stood so she could pull them down. She moved her mouth over his penis. He leaned over and touched her.

"Do you want to fuck me?" she asked.

"Yes."

She crawled onto the bed on all fours. Richard rolled on a condom and entered her. Bob picked up his video camera and started taping. Richard thought the couple seemed "normal enough," so he let the video roll. Tabitha went down on Richard while Bob watched. Then Richard entered her from behind. Tabitha started performing oral sex on her husband. Rather than stare at Bob's penis, Richard concentrated on what he was doing, on Tabitha's derriere, and the tattoo she had in the small of her back.

After both of the men climaxed, Tabitha and Richard cleaned up; they then sat and chatted for another twenty minutes. Tabitha wanted more, though. She wanted Richard to ejaculate on her breasts. She bent down to him. While she sucked on him, Bob entered her from the rear. When he finished, Richard still hadn't come, so he offered to do her again.

Richard started Tabitha on her hands and knees, before moving her flat on her stomach, and finally into the missionary position. Then she climbed on top and used a vibrator on her clitoris while Richard—to use his terminology—continued fucking her. He didn't come a second time, but he still thought it was great.

Minutes later, Richard was dressed, standing at the door, and asking the couple to send him a copy of the videotape. Bob refused—they'd have to exchange addresses and he wasn't comfortable with that.

The next day, Richard sent them a thank-you email offering to meet again.

. . . . .

"Tell me about sex, please," I posted on Craigslist Buffalo, New York.

"I was married for 10 years and I have a son (who lives out of state with his mother)," Richard answered. "I have a girlfriend now (and we are intimate), but I'm always looking for more on the side."

Richard was in the navy and stationed in San Diego, when we first started communicating, but he was born in Buffalo, hence his reason for searching the Buffalo casual encounters.

His girlfriend lived thirty minutes from him. Between the distance and her work hours, they only slept together once a week, at most. That's why he was looking for "some on the side." Plus, he explained, he wasn't very experienced before he got married. Despite the fact that he'd joined the military right out of high school, Richard didn't lose his virginity until he was twenty-four. He "was too naïve" to do it when he'd had the chances, he said, so now he was trying to make up for lost time. "I'm not married, not even engaged, so as long as I'm having safe sex, why not have as many partners as I can?" To accomplish that, he'd joined AdultFriendFinder.com, the self-proclaimed "World's Largest Sex & Swinger Personals" site.

By proper definition, swinging is for couples who have recreational sex with multiple consenting partners. However, singles often try to throw themselves into the sex mix, which might account for AFF's popularity; it doesn't limit its membership to couples. When Richard and I met, AFF had approximately 20 million members, with 70 percent of those being U.S. residents. Despite Richard's AFF membership, as well as memberships in so many sex/dating websites that he couldn't remember them all, Richard was shy.

I discovered that when I phoned him, which I did because, unlike Sean, Richard felt safe. He'd answered my email queries in a straightforward manner with no game playing or come-ons. He'd emailed me his phone number, we'd made an appointment, and I'd dialed at the appointed time.

Though he is shy, he likes to have Internet chat room sex, meaning he types what he would say and do to a woman while they're having sex as others in the chat room read along. Through one of those sex sites, he met a woman in his hometown of Buffalo.

"We were both just planning on meeting each other, and as long as we got along, jumping in the sack," he tells me. Instead, they sat in a bar and talked for three hours, followed by five minutes of kissing in the parking lot. "I was kind of hoping she'd invite me back, and I guess I would have gone with her that night." Rather, they made plans to see each other the next day at her house for some noontime sex.

As he drove to her house the following day, he wondered if she was going to rip off his clothes and he was just going to jump in bed with her. *How do we do this?* he thought.

When he got there, she said, "I'm not sure. How do we do this?"

"So we ended up sitting there and talking for another hour," he says. "Even though I'd like to have a kind of a no-strings-attached thing, I guess I need more than that. I need somebody that I get along with, somebody I'm interested in, somebody who's interested in me. That's why I guess I've never gone to a prostitute."

In truth, Richard has gone to a prostitute. It was after his divorce, with a woman he'd met on a website. "But I didn't realize at the time that she was a prostitute. . . ."

Richard, like many of the men I talked to, insists that countless women on the Internet dating sites are professionals posing as potential girlfriends in order to get paying clients.

"It was relatively inexpensive. And that's one of the reasons [I went to her]. I'm not gonna go out and spend a hundred bucks to get laid." The other reason was he was "just really horny."

"So I went over to her apartment, and we had sex. But it was— it really—uh, I wasn't attracted to her at all. I wish I hadn't done it. You know, I could have just as easily gone home and masturbated and would have felt just as good."

Richard then admits that he's on antidepressants that affect his sex drive. "Although I still get really horny . . . it's when it comes to masturbation, it's a little harder for me to come than it used to be. So now I need images, pictures, maybe porn movies, more than I did before." His preference is for anal sex porn.

Indeed, when he meets someone through an Internet sex chat

site—or a phone chat line—if the other person is a professional "escort," he always asks her if she does anal and if she has a nice ass. "I'm very attracted to that in a woman, more than anything else." He then inquires about her rates, what she's "into," and what she'll do—just to give himself "a little excitement." It's the taboo-factor that turns him on. But he never actually hires them.

* * * * *

Richard and I had our more than hour-long phone conversation weeks before he met Tabitha and Bob. About forty minutes into our conversation, I say, "Does AIDS, or any other kind of sexually transmitted diseases, concern you?"

"It does," he answers. "I don't use a condom with the girl I'm seeing now 'cause we discussed it beforehand." He hadn't had sex for the six months before they started dating, so he felt "pretty confident" that he was disease-free. "But if I ever had sex with anybody else, I'd definitely use protection just to be on the safe side."

Five minutes later, I begin closing our conversation and saying good-bye, when Richard clears his throat. Hesitantly, he interrupts me. "After I got a divorce and was having trouble meeting women, I found a, um . . . ," he stumbles over several syllables before finally saying, "gay Internet thing and hooked up with a guy. He gave me oral and then I had anal sex with him. . . . But he was the only guy I did it with."

That had been when Richard was stationed on the East Coast. In San Diego, his male-on-male sex life had escalated.

"I've hooked up with a lot of guys just to get oral sex because, um—I don't consider myself bi or gay. I still don't because I won't touch a guy's penis. I definitely wouldn't give him head or even jerk him off, but I figure, hey, if somebody wants to go down on me, I don't care if it's a man or woman. It all feels the same. I mean, in a lot of ways men are better at it because they kind of know what's going on. So I've probably had maybe ten different guys or so that I've met that have gone down on me."

He stops and clears his throat again. "A few of them have asked me to have anal sex with them, but I haven't. I've been thinking about it more and more, but, uh, again, I still don't consider myself bi because I'm not interested in guys that way. I'm just interested in the sex more or less. I thought you might find that part interesting."

I most certainly did. In fact, that had been on my list of questions for him: Have you ever had a same sex experience? But feeling as awkward about asking the question as he had been in telling me, I skipped it. So as I silently thank God for Richard's courage, I hear Richard say, "A blowjob's a blowjob, so why not?"

Still, I have to ask him why he went on a gay site in the first place. Richard clears his throat again. "I was doing it to meet women."

Huh?

In actuality, one night in San Diego, Richard had dialed up a phone sex chat line to meet women, when the automated instructions announced the options of men meeting men and women meeting women. "And I thought, huh, I didn't know there was one of those." For the hell of it, he says, he started listening. "It was the same thing, like I said. I was horny and not getting sex and was interested in getting a blowjob from somebody. . . ."

He was, in his words, "really, really nervous, you know. I'm still nervous now. . . . I don't feel as right about it when I'm done with that as having sex with a woman."

"Do you mean you're having guilt feelings?"

"Yeah, yeah, kinda. You know, a lot of times I'll get done and say, man, I'm never gonna do that again. And, a week later I want to again. But, yeah, there's a lot more guilt associated with that than with a woman."

"You think that's your Catholic upbringing?"

Richard practiced Catholicism until his parents divorced when he was ten years old.

"Um, I don't know. I don't think so, because I rarely think about that. I guess it's just the fact that, you know, I'm not gay and I'm not bi and just, you know, why am I doing this with a guy?" His voice turns low, embarrassed, and mumbling, so much so that his words are barely audible. "And I'll just kind of want to leave. So it's like, 'Well, thanks, but I've gotta go.'"

"Is there any kissing?"

"No," he answers. "I usually just kind of get undressed and, um, lay back on the bed or whatever and let 'em do whatever they want to do. But, no, like I said I don't—I'm not bi. I've never kissed a guy. I've never touched another man's penis. I don't—I would never want to. That just doesn't interest me in the slightest. But the physical aspect of having sex, you know, the blowjob, that does."

I ask if the other guy undressed.

"There's one or two that have. I don't particularly like it when they get undressed. And I definitely keep my eyes closed because I don't want to see a naked guy."

"I have a question for you," I say. "Since you have a thing for anal sex, and here are these gay men offering their rear ends to you, why not take them up—other than that once?"

"Um, why I haven't? I don't know. I guess maybe because," he stutters as he tries to get the words going, "when it's a woman's body and it's beautiful and, God, I just love women's bodies. And I just wouldn't feel the same if it was a man there, you know, with a hairy back or whatever."

What woman doesn't know?

"I just keep my eyes closed and concentrate on the sensations . . . but I try not to think about the fact that it's a guy any more than I have to."

"So you're keeping your eyes closed and visualizing a woman?"

"Yeah."

Most of Richard's encounters with men lasted less than twenty minutes. As he put it, "They come over and they suck me, I ejaculate, and they leave." The one exception was a gay massage therapist who Richard paid for a massage only. "But then it would just lead to him starting to jerk me off and then going down on me." Richard saw him, as well as one other man, perhaps as many as ten times each.

We talk on, with Richard repeatedly saying he isn't interested in men and he is with them only for the sex. If he were with a male-female couple, he says, he'd let the man touch him, but he still wouldn't touch the man. "I'd be just as happy with just the woman. But, you know, I'll put up with a guy if I have to, I guess is what I'm saying." He clears his throat.

By then, and as I listen to him repeat the same thought, I feel like I am hearing such hurt in his voice. Such guilt. Such longing. I want to comfort him. But my shrink warned me about getting too involved in my subjects' lives. I'd made that mistake before, and it had hurt my work, and it had hurt me. Besides, getting involved in your sources' lives isn't journalistically ethical. A journalist needs—must—keep a professional distance to report the story as objectively as humanly possible. I keep reminding myself of all of that.

"Richard," I say, and it is as though I stand in a tornado; it rips off my journalist's business suit, and I am sitting there just being Suzy the person, in my Levi's and sweatshirt, not Suzy the reporter. "This isn't my place to say this, but I'm going to say it anyway. Don't be ashamed. There's nothing wrong with it, and I'm—you're talking to a Southern Baptist here. But don't worry about it."

Just like Richard, I'd given in to the temptation. And just like him, I feel better and I feel worse for it. I love my Levi's and sweat-shirt, but I want the protection of my business suit, too.

"Well, I guess the only thing I really worry about is somebody finding out," he says. "Even though I'm straight, you know, people would go, 'No, you're not. You can't do that and be straight. You're bi. Or you're gay.' And I know I'm not. . . . The way I look at it I'm not. Maybe some other people would."

"But, I guess it's, you know, I'm nervous about it because I don't want to get caught. Other than that, I really don't care. It doesn't bother me that guys come over here and go down on me." He return to mumbling so quietly that again I can barely understand his words. "If anybody found out, I'd be too embarrassed to meet them face-to-face." He softly adds, "You've just gotta do what you gotta do."

Richard, too, had asked me for a photograph. But with him, it didn't feel like a sexual request at all, and I don't say that because he had sex with men. It just felt like pen-pal communication. Though I didn't send him a photo, I did let him know he could probably find a picture of me somewhere on the Internet. Richard didn't push me further.

Nor did I push him. I turned my attention to swinging.

∙ ∙ ∙ ∙ ∙

I'd studied swinging in college—at Baylor University, of all places, the largest Southern Baptist university in the nation.

One of my sociology textbooks back then was *Open Marriage* by married partners Nena O'Neill and George O'Neill. My 1973 paperback copy of the book describes this "new lifestyle for couples"—in essence, swinging—as "the O'Neills' exciting, original approach to married life."

The back cover refers to traditional marriage as a "stifling, limited arrangement" but says that it "can be opened up into an honest, undemanding, joyful relationship" through the *Open Marriage* concepts of "trust, liking, role flexibility, individual freedom and growth, and love and sex without jealousy," which could "do wonders for your marriage." The O'Neills, who later divorced, dedicated their book to each other.

Strangely enough, I don't recall being appalled by the concept of an open marriage. Maybe that's because I saw the book as just another textbook, so how could that reflect the real world? Or maybe it's because I couldn't relate to it. After all, I had no intention of ever getting married. I had sat in chapel, which was required at Baylor, and listened to preacher after preacher proclaim that a woman was like a rose who hadn't fully bloomed until she became a wife and godly mother as described in the Old Testament. She cooked, sewed, parented, gardened, taught, took care of business, took care of the poor, never slept, was always smiling and optimistic, and never caused her husband any trouble at all, says Proverbs 31. I focused instead on Matthew 19 in the New Testament, where Jesus says "it is better not to marry." He admits that not everyone can accept that idea due to a yearning for sex. It is only for "those to whom it has been given"—eunuchs.

"For there are eunuchs who were born that way from their mother's womb," Jesus says. "And there are eunuchs who were made eunuchs by men; and there are also eunuchs who made themselves eunuchs for the sake of the kingdom of heaven. He who is able to accept this, let him accept it."

I decided to accept that. To me, being a sexless eunuch, so to speak, seemed a lot easier than being a godly wife. Plus, from my reading, it seemed to me that being a eunuch was Jesus's first choice. And being a godly wife was Jesus's Plan B for those who were weak.

Still, the book *Open Marriage* obviously fascinated me. It's the only textbook I ever remember reading quickly. And I've kept my $1.95 copy so long that its pages aren't simply yellowed; they're oranged. So when I started researching swinging, I immediately knew where to find my copy of *Open Marriage*—on the bookshelf, top row to the right, in my bedroom at my mother's house, near my freshman year calculus book, a book I never comprehended until graduate school.

Similarly, I don't think I truly comprehended swinging. But I was going to.

Chapter 5

· · · · ·

On a ninety-degree Valentine's Day in Texas, Frank, a swing club owner, climbed into his white pickup truck and drove south on Interstate-35. About the same time, I jumped in my car and headed north on I-35 toward Waco.

Frank didn't know it, but I'd chosen our meeting place at a bookstore halfway between us because I knew a man who worked at the store and knew he'd look out for me if anything happened. I was a tad anxiety-ridden. This would be my first face-to-face interview with one of my sex sources. It had taken me more than two and a half months, the length of time since I'd posted my first Craigslist ad, to talk myself into it. But that wasn't unusual. I always have to psych myself into doing interviews, especially in-person ones. Even then I finally have to figuratively yell at myself, "Do it!" I'm not exactly a social human being.

So while still hiding behind my keyboard and monitor, I'd found Frank's club. It was listed on the website for NASCA International, known as the North American Swing Club Association before it went international.

Via NASCA and AFF, I quickly realized that Texas was second only to California in swinging population. (Florida was third, New York fourth).

· · · · ·

"I come from a strong Southern Baptist upbringing," Frank says as we sit outside the bookstore. His mother was his Sunday school teacher, his father a church deacon. And I'm staring at the hard-pack of Marlboro cigarettes tucked in the pocket of Frank's black, Tommy Bahama shirt, when, suddenly, he changes the subject. Then he changes it again. "I'm a little distracted right now." Just before leaving his house to meet me, he explains, he learned that a former girlfriend had died. She, like his wife, had died of cancer.

In fact, several years into Frank's only marriage—to a woman he describes as his soul mate—his wife was diagnosed with cervical cancer. She passed away just eighteen months before. That was one of the first things Frank told me when we talked on the phone to set up our interview.

"I like you," he says to me now, "so I just wanted to be honest with you. So if I seem like I'm a little out there . . . and not as quick, it's because I'm trying to figure out how to get to West Texas for a funeral."

Frank was born in New Mexico but moved to Texas with his mother after his parents divorced. "As I know you better, I'll tell you more. It's just me being protective over—my family. Do you mind if I smoke?"

I silently nod okay, despite the fact that I abhor cigarettes and am terribly allergic to tobacco smoke.

"Actually I was almost quit," Frank remarks as if reading me. "I was trying to quit, but I got a hospice counselor, you know, that's still with me and he said, 'The last thing you need to do right now is quit smoking.' I was quittin' for my wife. She had quit, and I was almost there. I'm trying to get past the stress of all of this, and

Valentine's Day is not the day for me to do it, you know . . ." His words float away with the smoke.

When Frank was eighteen years old, a former girlfriend—former because she'd cheated on him—told him she was pregnant with his child. They never married, but they did have a son. Two decades later, their son was killed in a hunting accident. Eight months after that, Frank's wife died.

"The problem with that is that I was so involved in my wife's care at that point that, you know, I didn't really get to mourn him as much as I'd like to because, you know," Frank speaks slowly and cautiously, "I'm not a hundred percent sure he is mine and not the other guy's. But it wasn't his fault . . . so I didn't feel any need to deny him what I could give him because of that."

Frank lights another cigarette. As his lighter clicks shut, he adds, "I don't normally chain smoke, but this is making me nervous. . . . I'm just not used to talking about this stuff. The only person who knew this stuff about me was my wife, probably. If you're looking for a reason for why I do what I do now, I don't think it's in there."

He is reading me too well. I am looking for a reason. He tells me that his parents never talked to him about sex, their divorce bothered him, he never got along with his stepfather, and because of his stepfather he moved out on his own before high school graduation, which resulted in Frank dropping out of school. He lost his virginity at age fifteen in the backseat of a 1969 Pontiac, to an "older woman" of eighteen. That was the first night his mother ever said to him, "Keep it in your pants," as he left for a date.

"Go figure that," Frank says, and he laughs.

He laughs a lot. He laughs when he describes that first sex. "It was short, okay." He has a smoker's laugh. "I can't believe I'm telling somebody this." He laughs some more with a big grin on his face.

Frank isn't the type of man I think of as particularly handsome.

He's just a nice-looking, average, middle-aged guy, but I can picture him as the dark bad boy that all the girls in high school wanted.

As if reading my mind again, he notes, "I'd say I had normal relationships through church and through school with different girls. Sex wasn't a big part of it. It wasn't like it's been my drive all my life. It's really not now. . . . I'm just very open-minded about it, okay."

He continues, "I'm pretty normal. I like two girls. What guy doesn't? . . . But with the exception of anybody hurtin' anybody or pedophilia or something like that, I'm not really judgmental about what other people do."

Thanks to Richard, I have the gumption to ask, and do ask, if Frank's ever had a homosexual experience.

Frank gets quiet.

Eventually, he starts to speak, hesitates, and stammers until he says, "I don't think it's influenced me in all this, but I was probably about thirteen. I had a man try something with me." Frank's words are deliberate. "It was a family member of a friend on a weekend trip away that tried to play with me in the middle of the night. . . . He tried, okay. He thought I was asleep, and I was too scared to do anything but roll over. But that's it. But I don't think that has anything to do with it."

By "it," Frank means his swinging lifestyle.

Frank didn't tell anyone about the attempted sexual abuse until years later. By then, the man had died. "And I was happy." Frank laughs uncomfortably. "I'm not a violent person, but that's one person I *loathe* the memory of."

Again, Frank emphasizes that that didn't influence the way he is. "I think the biggest influence on the way I am is—I just had the opportunity to do a few things that most guys just think about, okay. It doesn't make me a stud; it just makes me lucky, in some people's respect, at least."

In his younger days, Frank played in a bar band, which "lucked" him into a few threesomes. "I never thought I could do anything like that. Jesus."

Driving home from a gig one night, the band stopped at a convenience store. Frank walked over to the magazine rack, where he spotted and picked up a swingers magazine. *What the hell is this?* He bought the magazine, read it, and showed it to his live-in girlfriend.

He claims he showed it to her out of novelty, curiosity, carnival shock. "It wasn't any big deal." They then went on a road trip, and Frank noticed that his girlfriend had brought along the magazine.

"You know," she calmly said, "I've always fantasized about being with another woman. We ought to check some of this out."

"I didn't wreck the car," Frank jokes to me. But he did get them to a swing club. Not long after that, Frank opened his own off-premise club, meaning sex can't happen in the club—people go home or to motels to do that. Eleven years later, the club tallies nine thousand members, according to Frank.

"There is not a stereotype here," he states. "And most people who are in it, you'd never know it to see them. I mean, look at me. Do I look like what you thought was a typical swinger?"

I try not to stare at the gold chain that hangs around his neck—or at the gold medallion that hangs from it. They tangle in the dark hair that curls from his tanned copper chest, which is visible because his Tommy Bahama shirt is only partially buttoned. I don't want to say he *does* look like my vision of a swinger, so I answer, "I didn't know what to expect."

He insists that my mind has to have some kind of picture.

I dodge the question again by saying that from what I've seen on television, I have more of a picture of the women.

He nods in agreement. "They're wearing the slut wear"—skin-tight dresses that accentuate the nearly exposed breasts and almost reveal the vagina—and he remarks that I don't look like someone who would fit in his club.

I laugh and say that I don't expect so. I'm in my Levi's 501s.

"Some of the people that I see and meet, they don't look different," he counters. "They're not different."

When Frank and I talked on the phone to set up our meeting, he told me that three ordained ministers are members of his club. "They're just honest about what they've thought of." He teases, "You know you've thought about it."

I chuckle. I'm not about to reveal anything.

"I have doctors, lawyers, judges," he brags. "I have elected officials. And I won't say anything further than that, okay," and he laughs.

Frank proceeds to teach me some of the swing lifestyle terminology. "Want to party" means a couple wants to have sex. "Full swap" means the couple's sex play with others includes intercourse, and "soft swap" means there is no penetration, but there is oral sex . . . or only the women play. "Non-swap" means the couple doesn't participate, but they do like to watch others have sex. And every couple, Frank says, sets their own rules, such as whether they play separately or only in the same room.

"Most of us hate the word 'swingers.' I do."

Frank didn't have to tell me that today's practitioners prefer to be called "lifestylers." I already knew that from chatting on the phone with a NASCA representative, who was a swinger and former Los Angeles police officer.

"Or 'swappers,' 'wife-swappers,'" Frank continues. "I hate that because that seems to generalize one thing that only a certain percentage of people do." On any given night, he insists, 60 percent of the couples in his club go home the way they came—with each other only. "I've got couples that come to my club and I've known for years that have never played with another couple. They love the environment. They love the eroticism. They like to tease and the exhibitionism and the voyeurism."

I glance around us to make sure no one is eavesdropping, and then I ask him to describe the "totally erotic" fantasy of a swing club.

Frank drifts off for a moment to ponder my question, while I wonder over the intensity of my curiosity. It shakes me. Then his words are quick. "I think the most erotic thing about it is—just like with anybody else in the real world, [in a] normal dating situation— the anticipation, the wondering, the intrigue of the anticipation of what might happen. I think that's as much of a turn-on as the actual act."

Frank emphasizes that despite the fact that there are lifestylers who want to sleep with just anyone to rack up their numbers, who like group sex or orgies with as many as twenty people, that has never been his ideal. "I'm selective. I like my partners to be as well." His words are purposeful, yet tentative, as if he's thinking things through before speaking. "I like personalities and brains. A little more going on than just store-bought boobies." He releases a stream of cigarette smoke. "It ain't about fun with just anybody. It's about the right experiences."

He and his wife believed in making friends with someone before inviting her into their bedroom—*her* because the other person usually was another woman. On those rare occasions that they did invite a couple, their time getting to know each other took much longer. "I want to be comfortable with him before I let him have my most precious possession—for even a short period of time."

In his soul, if not in his actions, Frank is, by his own admission, personally and politically "very conservative." He sighs before adding that he isn't a conservative when it comes to someone legislating his morals. "I believe that's between me and my Lord and not for any politician to decide."

Me and my *Lord*. I'm stunned and taken aback by that phrase. I hear it in my brain over and over. *Me and* my *Lord*. That's when I ask Frank if he considers himself a Christian.

"I have trouble thinking all of this was an accident, okay, just because of the belief that I was raised with."

But Frank has a bit of difficulty responding to my question about how he meshes swinging with his Christianity.

"I don't know that I need—I'm not sure why the mesh—" He sputters as he considers his thoughts and words. "I don't believe there's quite the conflict there that the Moral Majority would have you believe, because in the Bible," again he stumbles around, "the rules regarding morality and sex were written for the man. A man can have a harem of wives, you know, multiple wives . . . and it's okay." Frank points out that women weren't allowed the same privilege, but he believes in equality—in both sexes being able to "enjoy life to its fullest" and having "a common bond with another person."

On the phone, Frank mentioned that swinging is sanctioned in the Bible. Though I wasn't so sure I agreed, I'd "uh-huh"-ed him at the time. Today I ask, "Is that in the Old Testament?"

He uh-hums a yes.

"Is there anything in the New Testament?"

"I'm not a theologian, okay, so I can't tell you that." His voice isn't defensive, only kind. "I just know that many, many large characters in the Bible had multiple partners or wives. But like I said, many women—I can't tell you exactly where you can find it—but in the Bible adultery is only a crime of women. I mean, did you ever read a Bible story that said *he* was stoned for committing adultery? And I think that's wrong. And I think that reflects the society and the people that were writing the scriptures more than I do the word of God, okay."

I'm not so sure I concur, but I keep that to myself. At Baylor, I'd made a D in Old Testament. I'd done only slightly better in New Testament—a rip-roaring C.

But Frank is right, I can't think of any men in the New Testament who were stoned for adultery, only for following Jesus. Then again, one of the Ten Commandments in the Old Testament is that thou shall not commit adultery. It doesn't say, "Women, thou shall not commit adultery, but, men, it's okay for you." The Ten Commandments also say don't work on the seventh day, the Sabbath. And I work almost every Sunday. So who am I to judge?

Frank lights another cigarette and reaches for his wallet. He pulls out a photograph of his wife. "Just a nice normal girl," he says. Sweat drips from his face. "To me, if there's a definition of evil, it's cancer. But, you know, cancer taught us both a lot. . . . It was a gift of sorts because it made us as close as two humans could be, you know, because we knew that tomorrow wasn't a guarantee. We had to live for the day with each other."

For three and a half years his wife fought her disease, and during that time, Frank didn't have sex with anyone else. "She told me I could do anything I wanted to do, but I didn't. . . . That wasn't where my head was at."

I ask him if he's had sex in the eighteen months since her death. "You don't have to answer that question," I apologize.

Frank is silent at length. Finally, he answers, "To a degree." He pauses for a beat as I chuckle. "Let's say I've been presidential. I've had presidential relief from close friends on a couple of occasions. . . . I've had much more offered, but I just, you know . . . I'm the only single guy that I know that regularly turns down invitations to orgies."

Then he stops and ponders again. "What I cry out for is—what my body wants right now is monogamy. And that makes sense because you want what you don't have or what you don't have access to, you know? I just want somebody to look at me with love in their eyes." He starts to light a cigarette. "Boy, that sounded corny."

"Doesn't everybody want that? Especially on Valentine's Day?"

"Yeah, this isn't my best holiday." We're both quiet, until he jokes, "At least I'm having a date with a girl." Then he lights another cigarette, his lighter clicking closed like a fast fade to black signaling the end of a poignant scene.

"Boy," I respond, "this is probably the best Valentine's Day I've had in—God knows—probably forever."

"Why?" he says.

Nervously I laugh. "I'm with a guy."

"Oh, you don't date anybody or anything?"

"No, nobody ever asks me out," I say. "I used to joke when I lived in L.A. that I could strip naked on Hollywood Boulevard and wave a thousand-dollar bill and say, here, come get me, the money is yours, and nobody would come up. I said that one night in a class, and there was this little, skinny, white guy who looked like he was a heroin addict, and he said, 'I'd take you up.' And I thought, Yeah, that's because you want the thousand dollars for the drugs."

I laugh hard.

I frequently make self-deprecating and probably inappropriate confessions in sexual situations. I'm not sure whether I do that to release the tension or to force a reassuring compliment. Maybe both. But if I were forced to guess, I'd lean toward the former.

Frank doesn't laugh with me, though. Instead, he says, "You've got the same confidence problems I have, obviously. You're a pretty lady. You shouldn't have that confidence problem."

I automatically laugh to cover my sudden discomfort. "Definitely," I chuckle. "Definitely." I immediately return the conversation to business. "I understand that when it's a threesome, the girl comes on to the other girl and then pulls the guy in." My bisexual friend Rose told me that. She's the one person I know who's had threesomes.

"Pretty much in this lifestyle, if they're doing it right, the women are in charge," Frank says. "Bi women is not the only thing in this lifestyle, but it is the catalyst for most of it. If something were to happen and all of a sudden there's a reason women don't want to be bi . . ."—perhaps a life-threatening STD that's passed only woman-to-woman, he suggests—"I'd be out of business. . . . There are some guys that really get off on seeing their wife with another man, but it's a very small minority."

With that, I want to know what happens in a swing club.

"I can show you that, okay," Frank says.

My stomach tightens.

"Play your cards right, I'll show you that, in a safe way."

My spine stiffens. But I hope that it's visible in my mind only and not in my body language.

Apparently it isn't, because all of a sudden, as if Frank senses my ill ease at his words, he stresses that he's very protective of his customers. "I don't go to the club at night thinking, Okay, what sex am I gonna have? And I didn't when I was married and we were involved in that."

Frank met his wife Angie over the Internet when they were chatting about how to download software. Their Internet chat moved to the telephone, where Angie asked Frank what he did for a living.

"How open-minded are you?" he replied.

Instantly she thought he owned a strip club. Frank explained, no, he owned a swing club. "I'm not looking for a swing partner. So that's not an obstacle," he quickly added.

"But she decided it was still okay to go out with me," he tells me. "And then our first real date was"—tears pool in the bottom rims of his eyes—"ten years ago today. I took her to Pizza Hut because the line was too long at the restaurants and took her to see *The Lion King*, which remained one of her favorite movies."

He weeps.

"I'm sorry," I say.

"It was a Thursday night. . . . I said, 'I'd like to see you again as soon as possible.' She said, 'Well, I have a date Saturday, so I can't see you then.'"

But Saturday morning, Angie phoned him. "I canceled my date. I'd rather be with you."

* * * * *

"The first time she walked into my club, she came in there with me, and, oh, I was nervous. I didn't put any expectations on her. I wanted her—whether she liked it or she didn't. As long as she accepted it, you know, the people, not so much as a participant, then that was fine with me."

The next weekend, Angie visited the club again. Upon returning from the restroom, she pointed to a woman and said, "That girl kissed me."

Frank asked, "Are you all right?"

"Yeah, I kind of liked it."

Two and a half months later, Frank proposed to Angie.

"And then we did our pillow talk thing about different ideas and fantasies and things like that. And one night with a couple of people I knew, friends of mine, she played with another girl." He pauses. "We never did anything when we weren't both in the room. We didn't have carte blanche to go off and party if we wanted, to go off and have an open marriage and an open lifestyle. . . . Some people do. We didn't."

"Tell me what I need to learn."

He thinks for a while. "I may have to do this with a few introductions. . . . I want you to come away from this knowing the caliber of people. . . . If I had to count on anybody in my world for something, I'd pick this group . . . because it's about friendship, not just sensuality and sex."

On the phone, Frank told me he couldn't have survived the past few years without the love and support of his lifestyle friends. Sex isn't the swinging prize, he stressed; the camaraderie of honest, open-minded people is. He pointed out that those same friends filled the church for his wife's funeral and that the preacher and Frank's family, neither of whom knows about his swing club, commented about what great friends he has.

But Frank grieves. "I feel myself these days kinda like persona non grata, but other people tell me different." Frank's referring to being a single man living and working in a couples-only lifestyle. Still, he's welcomed—even invited in—because people like him and say he fits in well. "I have trouble feeling like that sometimes," Frank continues, "but . . . I'm not perceived as a threat. I'm flattered about that, but it's not what I want to do, okay, you know." His voice becomes tinged with reluctance. "I don't know where I fall into in all of that. I'm still searching for my identity."

"Aren't we all," I say. "I just hit the big five-oh and am still desperately searching."

"I'm hittin' the four-five in two months, so I'm chasing you, darling. I'm a-chasing you."

"How about we knock this off and I take you over to buy you a Valentine's drink?" I don't ask Frank that because I want him to chase me. I ask him because I'm tired and want to stop and because he seems so sad on this Valentine's Day. I want to try to make him feel not so alone.

As Frank and I walk to a nearby T.G.I. Friday's, he hints that he wants me to turn off my recorder. A few minutes later, as we sit with our Valentine's margaritas and I'm without my recorder, I feel less safe. I realize that no one knows where I am. My friend who I'd hoped would look out for me at the bookstore wasn't there. I also remember that during my phone conversation with Frank, he mentioned that he was ready to start dating, that he'd seen my photograph on the Internet, and that he was already picking out clothes for me to wear at a swing convention held every summer in Las Vegas, that we could go together.

I just laughed at the time.

Now I'm sitting with him in the bar side of T.G.I. Friday's, which is maybe a notch or two above Pizza Hut, on Valentine's Day, which is the ten-year anniversary of his first date with his future wife, and sharing alcoholic beverages. On top of that, I feel he is asking me too many questions about me, like he is coming on to me. Then he pulls out of his pocket a dark wooden carving that he says he always carries with him. It's a small bust of his wife, but it looks more like a shrunken head. Maybe it's the true crime writer in me creating murder scenarios. All I know for certain is that it freaks me out. I want to leave. When we do leave, Frank walks me to my car, but I don't perceive his gesture as gentlemanly. I fear he's noting the make of car I drive and memorizing my license plate number so that he can learn where I live—the true crime writer again.

My worry was needless, though. Frank didn't follow me. Nor did he ever phone me. In fact, we never saw each other again. And I never went to his club. Part of me wishes I had gone . . . as that rare single woman who had enough guts to go by herself.

Chapter 6

· · · · ·

Frank consumed my thoughts, though, as did Richard, who'd discovered he had an STD, and Jim, Sean, Amanda, and the more than half dozen others who'd contacted me but soon disappeared. Of those who'd disappeared, some vanished because they only wanted a casual encounter, others faded because they realized they didn't really want to share the details of their sex lives. And I realized I didn't know what to think about this sex world I was tiptoeing around. I wondered how long it would take me to find the courage to actually set foot in it.

To some degree, it took me two weeks after sitting down with Frank. That's when I gutted up and joined Richard and Amanda and placed my own ad on AFF, as well as Alt.com, the self-proclaimed "World's Largest BDSM & Lifestyle Personals." (AFF and Alt are part of the same corporation.)

I put practically no personal information in my ads. No height. No weight. No eye color. No photograph. No nothing. I merely said I was looking for men, women, and couples to interview for a book. Apparently, any new, single female is a hot property who gets scores and scores of "views" and numerous "winks." My personal email box continually beeped telling me I had messages from AFF and Alt subscribers who were interested, though most were interested in doing things other than talking.

Dusty, a fifty-five-year-old rancher and Alt member in Texas, however, was willing to communicate.

"For years I had desires that were deeply sexual and I wanted to open up to my spouse about those needs," he wrote. "Finally I did and she did not understand. My choice was to either hide those desires or find some way to explore them." He did both—via the Internet, without his wife's knowledge. "I am heavily into anal play, enemas, wearing panties, oral sex, anal sex, both receiving and giving."

Dusty described himself as a university-educated man, successful enough in his own business that he retired before deciding to go into ranching. His Alt photograph depicted a distinguished, white-haired gentleman rancher—i.e., a typical boot-wearing Texan: tanned, clean-cut, part cowboy and part preppy.

Also characteristic of many middle-class baby boomer Texans, he was the son of yellow dog Democrats—meaning his parents would vote for an old yellow dog over a Republican—and he became a Republican. "I never paid attention to politics until I was in the military. I am a Vietnam veteran—the real kind, in country. I found that I was a hardcore Republican. Still am. Always will be. My family considers me a far right-winger. Yes, I own guns and carry one under a concealed handgun license, not because I need to, [but] because I have that right!"

"I know this sounds stupid, but should I be demanding in my questions?" I wrote, trying to be respectful of his desires. Besides wearing women's panties, Dusty liked to play submissive to a woman.

He laughed at my question. "I am as normal and sane as the next person, which may not mean much. LOL. Just ask me any way that meets your fancy."

Submission relaxed Dusty because he could give up control, he said. "Sometimes it is better to be told what to do. Does that go back to my military days? Who knows?" But he knew that it allowed him to enjoy pleasing others, which he loved to do.

Finding a compatible Dominant female partner, however, limited Dusty's submissive play. "I have found it very difficult to find people who understand and can share themselves to the degree that is required." Add to that the fact that many women won't play with married men, and that left Dusty talking with me, often a couple or more times a day.

"Sex with my wife . . . is basic and wonderful," he said. "We fully enjoy each other. Yes, I wish at times we could share more of my needs and desires, but I have learned to know that will not happen. I guess in a good deal of marriages the same would apply one way or another." He later added, "I hate secrets but my need is too great. Maybe God will forgive me for it. Maybe not." Dusty had been reared strict Catholic.

"I still consider myself a Catholic until this day I guess, but I do not practice my religion. Too many things have happened in the church—abuse, etc.—for me to be crazy about the organization, but I still feel that the religion itself is more true to my beliefs in a whole."

I guess I, too, will always consider myself a Southern Baptist, despite the fact that the Baptist church I grew up in isn't the same as the Baptist church of today. The Southern Baptist church of my youth taught love, grace, and mercy. Today, I hear shame, judgment, and condemnation, as though a forefinger is being shaken in my face and an index finger is being jabbed in my chest. I long for the church of my youth, but I didn't want to linger on my own religious hurt and disappointment.

My AFF mailbox was filling with invitations from men only. No women, no couples. The men inundated me with photographs of their penises, some erect, some flaccid, all unsolicited. I got so bored with these photos that I finally and rudely emailed one man that I'd respond when he came up with a more creative introduction than a photo of his penis. Not surprisingly, I never heard from him again.

In contrast, a gray-haired professional from the world of high-tech had posted a golfing shot of himself on AFF. Standing on the course, a club in one hand and dressed in all-black golf clothes, he had a somewhat nouveau riche aura about him that would allow a lot of women to ignore his senior citizen paunch. He emailed me a few times, but before our correspondence reached each other, he'd replaced his demure golf shot with a picture of his penis. I wanted to know why he'd changed the photo, why men sent women pictures of their penises, and whether such photos worked.

At first, he responded politely that the golf picture was still there, along with others; he just regularly rotated his photos. Then he firmly stated that in the two years he'd been an AFF member, his G-rated pictures had gotten zero response. If he contacted a woman who had posted a nude picture of herself, the first thing she wanted from him was a picture of his "equipment" since people on the site were there "looking for sex." As proof that his penis photo worked, he quoted a woman who'd given him what he called a "testimonial"— "I would Love [sic] the opportunity to feel your balls in my hand rise when your huge cock begins pulsating in my mouth as I suck hard to get that last sweet droplet of cum out of you as it flows smoothly down my throat."

Next, he specifically declared to me, "That is not because I was holding a golf club."

Mr. Golfer never said whether he actually met with the writer of his testimonial, nor whether she was one of the alleged sex professionals on the site posing as a potential girlfriend in order to find clients, or whether she was one of the ones who like to flirt vicariously but never show up for a meeting.

Instead, thirty-six minutes later he emailed me, "Sex between people is only when it's desired by all parties; sex begins in the mind and then builds to the physical touching, kissing, hugging, and finely

[sic] the intimate act itself. In this case you have stimulated me as much as a cold shower so at this point the chances of me having sex with you are slim and slimmer.

"Please don't think I changed pictures for you, I have 20 women in my network that really want to get laid and some for the second time so please don't think that was done for you, it was not!"

Shaken, I emailed my friend Rose. "Some 'multimillionaire'"— or at least he claimed to be a multimillionaire—"got ticked at me, I guess because I was telling him the truth about writing a book and he wanted to play like it was fantasy, I guess. Anyway, he got rude and was a jerk. And it upset me."

So I turned my attention to a man who called himself Sadistic Bastard. Sadistic Bastard and I had met through Craigslist. He was a forty-five-year-old Dominant who had been in the BDSM— bondage and discipline, dominance and submission, sadism and masochism—lifestyle for twenty-eight years.

BDSM had always given me the heebie-jeebies. I'd turned down a true crime book offer years before just because the murders had involved BDSM; I didn't think I could psychologically handle the topic. Sadistic Bastard's polite one-paragraph email offering his help had tensed the muscles in my elbows and made my neck twinge with angst. But unlike so many other men I'd heard from—men who weren't into BDSM—Sadistic Bastard was the utmost gentle-man, even gallant, to the point of asking me how I preferred to be addressed. He said he was the son of a career military officer. He'd discovered the "Lifestyle," as he called BDSM, when he was in high school.

"The terms D/s and BD/SM have only been around for the past fifteen years or so," he wrote.

D referred to Dominant; s referred to submissive or slave. I eventually learned that the Dominant is always capitalized and the s is always lowercased because of its submissive status to the Dominant.

"Yet, the Lifestyle can be traced back through the history of Europe and even further back in Eastern cultures," he explained.

Sadistic Bastard regularly gave BDSM lectures and demonstrations. "There is one thing to keep in mind when talking with those in the D/s and BD/SM Lifestyle. No two people are the same. With that said, the same holds true to Lifestyle Groups and Organizations. Each is different, with its own views. Nothing is written in stone. Yet there are many general rules and views that are shared by most people in the Lifestyle. These protocols are handed down from generation to generation, with each adding to them or removing to suit their own needs."

Though one could easily get involved in the Lifestyle today by searching the Internet, Sadistic Bastard said when he discovered BDSM in the 1970s there were only two ways to get involved: "One, you went looking for it or, two, the Lifestyle came and found you, meaning someone in the Lifestyle thought you had the personality and the right makeup to enjoy or do well within the Lifestyle."

Just as there had been two ways to get involved, there were two types of Dominants, too. "One is a Dominant by nature and the other is a Dominant by nurture, meaning a person can be taught to be in the Dominant role. I know there are many CEOs of major companies that in their private lives are submissive and that this submissive role is their true nature. Yet they were taught to take on the Dominant role in the business world."

I felt a bit overwhelmed. Talking with someone named Sadistic Bastard. Talking about having a personality to dominate someone, to hurt them, to control them, with rules but without rules. I knew I had too much to learn. Could I handle it?

To be honest, I couldn't. I kept thinking about that BDSM true crime I'd refused to write. The women who had been murdered would probably still be alive if they hadn't been involved in BDSM. I had to remove myself for a while. I didn't communicate with Sadistic Bastard again until I'd had so many AFF men be so rude to me that I longed for his courteous ways. That was nearly three months after he and I had first met through the Internet, the same way those BDSM-loving women had met their killer.

• • • • •

Sadistic Bastard specifically instructed me to phone him. "Not because of the bill on the phone," he explained. "It is just one of the safety practices I preach to women about giving out their phone numbers to people they meet on the net."

When I do call him, the rudeness of the male swingers from AFF and the kindness of Dusty from Alt are on my mind. So the first thing I say to Sadistic Bastard is "I'm finding that the people at Alt .com are much nicer than the swingers, so to speak. Is that a total generalization on my part?"

He chuckles lightly. "When you speak nowadays of alternate lifestyles, this is a huge umbrella. It's grown to incorporate so many different things. And swingers compared to what they call Lifestylers are like comparing zebras to horses. You know, they both kind of look alike, but they're two different animals."

To Sadistic Bastard, "Lifestylers" solely means BDSMers, not swingers. In fact, I was beginning to believe that swingers had stolen the "lifestyle" moniker from the BDSMers.

"So much about what is considered the Lifestyle is based upon respect. You're dealing with people that are very—especially when you're dealing with Dominants that are very aggressive, assertive, you can feel very easily threatened. So it's kind of like a mutual respect kind of thing, you know. You don't push my buttons, I won't push yours kind of thing. And swingers aren't like that. They're, you know, they're in it for the [sex] ride."

"So I'm not totally wrong?" I ask, feeling so very naïve.

"No, no, you're not. You're pretty much correct. But then again, you know, this is a generalization. For every rule there is an exception."

"And I'm hoping to find that exception because I know there's got to be some nice swingers out there," I say.

Just as the Internet has altered the world of swinging—"fueled it right up through the roof," as one swinger described it to me—the Internet has changed BDSM. Sadistic Bastard points out that without the Internet, I never would have found the BDSM underground. "We don't wear signs," he laughs.

He is the eldest of five children, and his career military father was a West Pointer, promoted to general. "He served all the way to his first star," Sadistic Bastard states with what seems to be a mixture of pride and remorse. "Everybody in my father's household was submissive. It's not that he ran his house with an iron fist. I mean, he wasn't—well, his favorite line was 'You have somehow come under the misunderstanding that this house is a democracy. It is not. It is a dictatorship.'"

Sadistic Bastard emphasizes to me that his father wasn't really a dictator. He just believed in his way or no way. But in high school, the future SB discovered there was another way when he dated an older woman who liked to be tied up, affording him his first opportunity to take on a Dominant role. It was, he says, "Whoo-hoo! Freedom at last!"

After high school, he joined the army, where he found other people involved in BDSM. "So I had quite a taste for it by the time I got out of the service." By then, he'd ruined every love relationship he'd had, he says, because he didn't know what he was doing when the relationship moved beyond sex. "To tie somebody up and have sex with them—have rough sex, have kinky sex, whatever—that is easy to do. . . . Being a Dominant away from the sex, now that's where it gets difficult, you know."

Like a child, a submissive might act up to get attention, he explains. But Sadistic Bastard didn't understand or realize that back then. "And I'd let my Irish temper go. It's not that I would throw things or hit them or something like that. I'd just throw them out of the house.

"So this is what I mean by screwing up. I wasn't giving them what they needed as far as the D/s went. So that's when I went out looking. And fortunately, at the time, I was in the northern Virginia area, which put D.C. at my fingertips. And back in the seventies, if you couldn't find it in Georgetown, it couldn't be found." That's where SB found the friends who taught him "the meaning of what the Lifestyle was about at the time." Then he was accepted into a group that provided him his first formal BDSM training.

And with that, Sadistic Bastard begins my education in the basics of BDSM. "In a relationship you have what is called a Master in the Lifestyle, and the submissive or the slave." He clarifies that Master isn't just a relationship; it is an earned title requiring certain learned skills, just like those of a master carpenter or a master plumber. In fact, there is a hierarchy of earned titles for Dominants— Sir, Dominant, Master, and finally Lord.

Today those rankings—and even formal training—aren't as predominant, or meaningful, as they were in the 1970s and "that there in itself is because of the Internet. Any Joe Schmo can put Master in front of his name and go and pretend to be somebody." Sadistic Bastard calls these Internet newcomers "fakes, wannabes, players."

"When I came into the Lifestyle, it was kinda on the cusp. It was going through a change." Fetish clubs and swing clubs were opening. The term "sadomasochism" was being replaced by "BDSM." And there was a mingling of doctrines.

"What do you mean?" I ask.

"You have different doctrines, as I refer to them. You have leather, which I'm sure you've heard the term before."

In the 1980s, I'd known of a gay professor who was into the "leather" Lifestyle. But in my ignorance, I'd thought that had meant he wore leather all the time to show off his muscles and hung out with other guys who wore leather all the time to show off their muscles—just like, in my mind, the carpenter from the Village People hung out with other guys in flannel work shirts and blue jeans.

I certainly was unaware for a thirty-two-year-old who had lived in New York City and Los Angeles.

"And there's old guard leather and then there's the Celtics and there's the House of Black Rose, and there's different doctrines out there that have different philosophies and beliefs."

"I guess I need to bone up on all of that," I say.

"Um," Sadistic Bastard moans doubtfully. "Some of that's going to be pretty hard to find, to be quite truthful. Like I said, even though the Internet has expanded everything and shed light on it and given access to every Tom, Dick, and Harry out there, there are still the hard-core Lifestylers. They're still pretty much underground." In fact, he says, they are *very* underground. "These people really don't associate with anybody but themselves. They go to national events and stuff. Like anybody else, they have friends from coast to coast that they associate with. But they're under the radar and they prefer to stay that way."

"Why is that?"

"Um . . ." He hesitates again. "Have you heard the term 'vanilla' yet?"

"I've heard it, but I don't know what it means."

"Okay, you have Lifestylers and you have vanilla."

"That's just plain ole people like me," I say.

"The rest of the world. There's us, and then there's them."

"Okay."

"So the vanilla world really doesn't choose to accept us. And they can do a lot of harm to someone's life, just because of the practices we have. . . . You could lose your kids. You could lose your business. There's so much you have to lose once society gets ahold of this information. . . . So these people are skittish of who they let know what, why, when, and where. You know, and there's things that they won't discuss."

"Do you consider yourself hard-core?"

"Yeah."

"So why are you talking to me?"

"My kids are grown. They are in college. I have less to lose."

He then explains that men and women in the BDSM Lifestyle have nicknames, or user names, that they use when playing—like Sadistic Bastard. "And I would say probably in the last seven years or so that I have stopped using my nickname and have started using my name, Patrick."

"Just because you have less to lose?"

"There was a time that, you know, when what our children did reflected on us. So it's not just what you can lose, it's the face that your parents or aunts and uncles and grandparents or whoever can lose, the embarrassment you can be to the family."

Oh, Lord, how many times had my mother told me, "How can you embarrass me like this?" whenever I didn't do what she wanted me to do, which usually involved seeing my uncle. And that was when I was in my twenties.

"It's the parents' fault that Junior does this. But . . . six, seven years ago, there was a point that it was kind of like, okay, I'm tired of hiding. I've been doing this too damned long, ducking, running, and staying under the radar, and I'm getting tired. You know, this is who I am and this is what I am, take it or leave it. So like I said, I've less to lose. . . ."

Patrick's a divorced engineer who has owned several companies.

"Have you heard the term power-exchange?" he says. "Power-exchange isn't necessarily considered BDSM per se." Whereas in BDSM there are Dominants and submissives or slaves, in power-exchange, there are tops and bottoms. "Someone is in charge or someone is giving and someone is receiving. It's kind of like a pitcher and a catcher playing catch. The pitcher would be considered the top and the catcher would be considered the bottom, even though the catcher is throwing the ball."

So I ask Patrick what's involved in a hard-core, 24/7 BDSM Lifestyle.

He gives me a "for instance."

"A Dominant or the Master would come home and his submissive would be butt-ass naked kneeling in the middle of the living room floor with nothing but a leather collar around her neck and her leather wrist cuffs and ankle cuffs. . . . Every day of the week when he came home from work, that's where she would be—or where he would be [if the woman were the Dominant]. It's very ritualistic. . . . The submissive does not sit on furniture. They'll kneel on the floor at their Master's feet. And if he were nice, he'd give them a pillow to kneel on because they're going to be there a while. You know, if he's watching six or seven hours of television, hardwood floor can be kind of hard on the knees. It's rough."

"So is that how you lived?" I say, but my voice sounds like that of a little girl.

"Yeah."

Quickly, I dig deep to find the reporter in me again, and in my business voice I say, "So what kind of woman is attracted to this?"

"This is where the vanilla world has a strange understanding," he says. "They think a submissive and a slave is someone that is weak-minded, weak-willed, and has no ambition. And that could not be any farther from the truth."

"Oh, yeah," I respond. "Part of me can see that, because you'd have to have a desire for it to stick with it. And that kind of ambition."

"Yeah. Well, here's the deal," he says. "The biggest thing in the relationship—" He stops and asks if I'm in a relationship right now.

"No, I'm not."

"Okay. Have you had any long-term relationships?"

"No," I laugh.

"How old are you?"

"Fifty."

"You're fifty? You've never had—What's the longest relationship that you've ever had?"

"Uh, six months. And we lived in separate cities." I'm still laughing. "I don't do relationships well."

Boy, that's an understatement.

"Okay. But still, even with yourself, you've had friends that have had long-term relationships?"

"Uh-huh."

"Okay. In your own relationships, and in their relationships, on a scale from zero to ten, where would you place trust? With zero being the least and ten being the most. You would put ten as the most important thing?"

"For trust, yes."

"Okay."

"So that's what this is, huh?" I say.

"Well, here's where it might surprise you. Okay. If you trust somebody at the level of ten, what you're telling me is that if this person told you to go stand on the roof of the house and jump, and he would catch you, that you would do it because you trust him that much. All right? Now you stand in front of somebody that's got a single-tail whip, this thing has the power, a bullwhip can take the hide right off of you, and it can lay a gash in you eight, nine inches long, three inches deep. It will rip through muscle. You know when a bullwhip cracks?"

"Oh, yeah," I say. I didn't grow up in Texas for nothing.

"And you know what makes that sound? . . . It is the end of that whip breaking the sound barrier. That's how fast the end of that whip is traveling. Imagine leather coming at you with the speed of sound. It will go through you like a bullet. You better trust somebody before you go stand up in front of them with a single-tail whip."

He reels off the names of several TV shows from the 1950s and '60s—*Ozzie & Harriet*, *The Donna Reed Show*, *Leave It to Beaver*, and finally *Father Knows Best*—and points to their marriages. "Happy marriages," he says, "long-term, but when you really get down to it that level of trust that they have in each other is below five.

"In this Lifestyle that trust level is up between seven and ten. It is the most important thing that there is in the relationship. Above everything else. I mean, what person would not want that—their significant other—that the trust that you have in them be the most important thing in their lives."

"Okay," I say, "for role-playing and everything, fine. But for me,

'Honey, I don't want to sit on my knees for twelve hours. I'm out of here. We'll do it later.'" Again I'm laughing. "It wouldn't be a matter of lack of trust. I just wouldn't want to sit on my knees forever."

"Well, I understand that," he answers. "We're trying to get into some of the mind-sets of people—that the trust that you have in somebody is that important, all right? And this is one of the things that pulls them into it. Another thing, you get into the characteristics that the vanilla world sees as weak-minded and weak-willed— have you ever seen that little game where they have one person stand, cross their arms across their chest, close their eyes, and fall backwards, and somebody catches them?"

"Right." I've always refused to play that game.

"Okay," he says, "the person that is falling back is the submissive or the slave. The person catching is the Dominant. Now between those two individuals in that scenario, who's stronger?"

"I guess the slave is what you're saying?"

"Yeah. Submissives and slaves always are going to be stronger than a Dominant. They're the stronger of the two."

"Because . . . ," I say. "I'm still not following why that would be the stronger one."

"Because of what they have to do to trust."

"Okay," I respond, still not sure I believe.

So Patrick continues. "Imagine the self-will that you have to have to do that—how much willpower. These submissives, men and women alike, are not weak-willed. They're not weak-minded. And they're not stupid."

This is all a little too intense for me. I can't get the sound of the speed-snapping bullwhip out of my head, much less the ripped hide, the deep bleeding gash well more than half a foot long. "Well, I think you just hit it that I'd be a Dominant," I say chuckling, probably nervously.

"You know, we all have personality traits," he says. "We're either Dominants or we're submissives. We're leaders or we're followers. Even in the vanilla world, you know. Some just choose to act a little bit more on it. Some just like to take it a little bit further to the extreme. When you get into kneeling and stuff—this is all very ritualistic. This is, you know, showing homage. It's showing respect. It's showing devotion.

"Do you know what a Saint Andrew's cross is? It looks like a big X. It's not like what you see in the Catholic church. Or what normally people wear around their neck. A Saint Andrew's cross is used for what's called scene-ing. Scene-ing is nothing more than just a fancy word for playing."

He asks if I know what a flogger is.

I knew it was some sort of whip.

"It's usually made of leather, in general terms, but it can be made with anything, rubber or string or anything else, but it has a lot of them. Not like a cat-o'-nine-tails. . . . But anyway, here's a scenario for you. Saint Andrew's cross, submissive, Dominant, flogger. Mind-set: The submissive or slave is strapped to the cross. They are tied. They're attached. They're restrained.

"This is where you are getting into trust issues. Okay. You're getting fear going. You're getting trust going. And basically what is being demonstrated is 'Master, this is what I will take from you.'

"You know what a safe word is?" he asks, not really waiting for an answer. "The most common safe words out there are red and yellow. Red means stop. Yellow means slow down. So . . . they know they've got a safe word, but, still, 'This is what I'll take.' This is the mind-set that they're in. 'I'm trusting you.'

"Now, same scenario, except for this time the submissive or slave is just standing there with their hands on it. They're not attached. They're not restrained. This is more of a mind-set of, 'Okay, I'm demonstrating my devotion to you. I will willingly stand here and let you flog me. . . .' You've got all the same things, but just changing it, altering it a little bit, you create a whole different scene in the mind-set of both of the individuals."

I seemingly change the subject. "Do you have to take classes on all this?"

"You are taught how to use a single tail. You are taught how to use a flogger. You are taught how to use a cane. All this stuff—have you heard the phrase 'safe, sane, and consensual'? SSC? Unt-uh!" he pronounces. "None of this is safe, sane, or consensual. I mean it's consensual. But . . . look at it. We're nuts. I'm the first one to admit it. There is nothing that I do in this Lifestyle that in any possible way would be considered sane by definition of the word 'sane.' There is nothing that I do that would be considered safe. You want safety? Sure, don't stand in front of me with a whip in my hand."

I don't see that being a problem for me, I think. But what I say is "Is this the same type of person who would be an adrenaline junkie jumping off cliffs?"

"I am an adrenaline junkie. Yes, I'm a retired base jumper. But, yeah, you've got the chemical reaction to go off in the brain that's different for the submissive and it's different for the Dominant, but still these things are going off."

"It seems to me that'd it be kind of a high."

"Yeah, there is a high to it. For a Dominant, most of the time, for me personally, and also in general terms, when you're scene-ing with a submissive or a slave, I'm getting out there on the edge. I'm getting very, very close to my primal instincts. Now, the trick is how close to that edge can I get and not fall off. We are all capable of doing the most horrendous things to human beings. The only thing that keeps me different from Mussolini and Hitler is the fact that I keep it in check."

He says the same thing goes for me—I just keep my primal nature in check when dealing with society. Then he adds that the phrase "safe, sane, and consensual" was created for the vanilla world, as a defense. "If we ever got dragged into court, if we were going to explain ourselves, [we'd say] this is all safe, sane, and consensual. I don't know of a jury in the world that would ever consider standing in front of somebody with a bullwhip as safe or even sane. Not unless you were in front of a jury of Lifestylers."

At that, I am *completely* overwhelmed. I'm freaked out. I'm emotionally spent. I absolutely cannot take anymore. But instead of saying that, I say, "Can we talk again, because I've got to absorb all of this . . . because this is just fascinating and so educational and I'm blown away by all that you've told me. And I mean blown away in a good way."

Chapter 7

· · · · ·

There were many reasons I was freaked out by my conversation with Sadistic Bastard. But there was one phrase of his that shook this true crime writer's brain so madly that its vibrations disturbed my body and my heart. "If we ever got dragged into court . . ." Those seven words kept me thinking about that book contract I'd turned down. It was the true story of a serial killer who met his female victims through BDSM websites, lured them into an in-person meeting, killed them, and stuffed their bodies in steel barrels, some of which he sank in the bottom of a lake, where they rotted. I could not imagine spending six months—the length of time it takes to research and write a paperback true crime book—in the black world of BDSM.

I couldn't fathom then or now why any woman would desire to be beaten, why she would seek it out, and why any woman—any person—would find it pleasurable.

"Man, this hardcore BDSM is seriously freaky shit," I emailed Rose.

But let me state now, I did not think—*not* at all—that Patrick, aka Sadistic Bastard, was a murderer. Quite the contrary. When I'd mentioned to him the possibility of meeting in person, he'd seemed reluctant before emphasizing that any such meeting would have to be a in very public place with others around us, not just for my safety, but his, too.

And when I'd told Patrick that I was blown away in a good way by what he'd said, I hadn't been lying to him. I'd meant that it was good information for the book.

Patrick had told me, "You talk to people that are in the Lifestyle, and especially the hard-core, and even the not so hard-core, that are into the D/s . . . and BD—bondage discipline and sadomasochism— and they will all tell you that . . . the involvement of sex in it all is less than fifteen percent of what we are and what we're doing. But why is a sexual act—eighty to ninety percent of the time—our first involvement in it?"

That, Patrick said, was something he'd been struggling with for the past several years—why sex was the first involvement.

But what kept tumbling through my mind was the 15 percent. I turned to Dusty and wondered in writing if what Patrick had said was true—that sex is just a small percentage of the Lifestyle.

"I get sexual satisfaction from being submissive to a woman," Dusty responded. "I have been with some that no sex is involved except for me being able to masturbate myself. Others do it for me. Some even go so far as the actual sex act. Trust me, when a woman takes you anally with a strap-on, it's sex.

"Now all that sounds as though I have been with many women, but in truth we are talking three encounters. I have had a few phone sessions as well and I think those could be classified as sexual.

"To the point, I guess it depends on the people involved whether it is sexual or not. For me, it is very sexual."

But nosey, curious me, I wanted to know specifics—the details.

"Okay, specifics about three encounters," Dusty returned. "Oh boy, this is gonna be a little harder. . . ."

First encounter was with a very nice attractive "femdom." She was a nurse and loved to play with a "submissive." She wanted me to be a "slut." She always had me wear sexy panties. She loved to give me multiple enemas that consisted of solutions of her choosing. The only sexual contact was her preparing me for the enemas, lube, etc. and her use of a strap-on on me anally. The strap-on was made so it was also inserted in her vagina. I am sorry if I am being too blunt on what happened. Not sure what detail you are looking for. When she was finished with my backside, she would watch me masturbate to climax. I never touched her sexually, and she would remain dressed in panties and bra except when using the strap-on. She was nude from the waist down during that.

The second encounter was much the same except there were two femdoms. They both took turns, again with me in panties, giving me enemas and playing with my anal area. Then one of the two, not both, had me lay on my back and she then got on me using a strap-on. She had my legs up in the air and screwed me for at least 20 minutes. She said it was her favorite way to use a man. They also enjoyed some cock and ball torture, and we did that as well. Both suggested they spank me, and I let them paddle me some.

At the end of that session, they both placed a condom on me with some type of warm lube that felt very nice and stroked me until I came.

The third encounter was with a lady that wanted to learn enema play. We met at a hotel, and I gave her a series of enemas. We played anal games. And then she gave me enemas. At the end of that session, she wanted me to have sex with her, vaginal, and we did.

Oh, I did have another encounter with a lady where we shared toys, enemas, and anal, oral and vaginal sex. That was a number of years ago, about three, and that was not so much of a submissive encounter but more of just sexual.

How did I feel? Wonderful. I love to give myself to someone and enjoy with them the things they enjoy and the things I do as well. It would not be fair to say I felt no guilt, as I am a normal human being. I just need the pleasure of giving so bad I cannot help myself.

I met all three through Alt.com. We exchanged email, and when they were comfortable about meeting, we chose a place that was public. All the encounters started at a place where we had lunch first and then agreed on playing. In the emails, we all researched likes, dislikes and boundaries, so they were agreed upon prior to even meeting.

. . . On average, the encounters lasted from three to four hours. The time spent is all a matter of schedules, etc. In one we laid in bed and talked longer than we played. We both really enjoyed just the openness we could have after what we had experienced with each other! Trust me, after a session like we have, it is one, if not the most, intimate things you would ever do.

As I learned more about Dusty, my mood darkened. He wrote that his father had physically abused him until he was fifteen years old. "My mother knew what was going on, but back then that type of punishment was considered okay, I guess." And I wondered if there was more at work than happenstance when he chose a nurse to give him enemas—his mother had been a nurse.

Dusty admitted that his childhood did influence his sex life, causing it to become a driving force in his life. "I loved it because it made me feel close to someone. I never got that at home."

· · · · ·

Suddenly, I was beginning to see a connecting thread in BDSMers, particularly the men involved in the kink Lifestyle. They all seemed to have been emotionally, physically, or sexually abused by their fathers—at least the ones with whom I'd communicated. So I started quizzing several shrinks about that. Some said, yes, it's true; most

BDSMers have been abused. Others said, absolutely no, it's not true. But no matter what the fact, for the first time in my life I was realizing how important a father is to a child, including a child's sexual development.

I know that sounds silly considering how many studies have been conducted on the importance of fathers, but I didn't have a father when I was growing up. He died when I was five. Although some people might consider that a loss—and I think some people in our church thought it was a sin that my mother never remarried—I believe it was a blessing from God because I had the privilege of being reared without the confinement of male/female roles.

In my family, my mother did everything—the cooking, the sewing, the minor plumbing repairs, the yard work, the making of the money, the budgeting, the investing, the saving for college and emergencies. She actually fulfilled the Old Testament description of a godly woman. And seeing how a woman could do anything and everything taught me to be ambitious, independent, and fearless. I could do and accomplish anything that God put in my heart, and I didn't need a man to do it, no matter what they taught me at Baylor and no matter how many sermons I heard about women and the necessity of men and children.

I just never realized how not having a father might have stunted me in my sexual development and sexual maturity.

· · · · ·

"I'm still reeling a bit from this sex research," I emailed Rose. I did okay in the daytime. It was the nighttime, the angry, penis-picture-sending men who crossed boundaries, and the Masters who did me in. "I mean, I can handle the gentlemen who are into *serious* BDSM, if"—that was the key word, *if*—"I don't think about them in their leather masks with their bullwhips ripping six-inch gashes into their slaves."

No, Sadistic Bastard hadn't said six-inch gashes. He'd said a bullwhip traveling faster than the speed of sound, laying in a nine-inch gash, three inches deep, that ripped off one's hide. I could see it in my mind—his black leather hood, a woman kneeling before him, naked, cowering on the ground, her arms and legs bound in thick restraints, the bullwhip cracking, the blood dripping. "Oh, I wish I could get this out of my brain."

I needed Doris Day–type sex in my head. *Sex and the City*–type sex in my head. Not dark, skin-slashing sex.

· · · · ·

Dusty seemingly read my need for some normalcy. He emailed me "a day in the life of a regular guy like myself."

Every day, Dusty rose around four-thirty in the morning and then sat on his porch while he drank two cups of coffee and thought about what he had to do that day. "If it is a day I go to my office in town, usually Monday through Friday, I shower, get dressed, etc. and go attack the problems associated with running a business. . . .

"If it is a day on the ranch, it's shower and dress, go plow, mow, haul hay, etc. . . . very relaxing and enjoyable except when the weather is rough."

On weekends, he often washed dishes, bussed tables, cooked, did anything that needed to be done to a help a couple of friends who owned a small family restaurant.

"They have a daughter, unmarried, who has three children, six, three, and two months. They think of me as a grandfather. In fact, this last weekend the two month old stayed the night with us as she wanted to go out.

"So what else about me? Hmmmmm . . . I sometimes do things for others to the point I do not have time to do what I need to do."

· · · · ·

I sat in silence as I thought about his words. I pictured him on the porch with his coffee, riding his tractor, sweat dripping from his brow, bussing tables with a white apron tied at his waist. I dreamed of going to that restaurant and watching him, visiting with him, laughing. But that didn't happen.

My mother fell and broke her hip, causing me to be away from my research. Suddenly, my sex freaks, as I had begun calling them, the handful of ones—like Dusty—who had been staying in touch with me on an almost daily basis, started inundating me with emails, wondering where I was and why they hadn't heard from me. They said they missed me and were concerned about me. Once I explained why I had been Internet silent, they responded with thoughts, prayers, and even words of advice as to how to help someone who is recovering from a hip fracture and surgery. With that, I began to preface the words "my sex freaks" with "the people I lovingly refer to"—as in "the people I lovingly refer to as my sex freaks."

Though I did try to write at the hospital, I had difficulty doing so. I feared my family would lean over my shoulder to read what I was typing. I knew they would be disgusted, to say the least, by the things my dear sex freaks were doing and, worse, would be fearful for me and what I was being exposed to. They would use words like "sick," "evil," and maybe even "Satanic" to describe the sex. And my family would worry, while praying more for me than for my mother, that I would be pulled into the burning clutches of the devil.

I didn't want that for them or me, and especially not for my mother.

And in so many ways, my sex freaks were so very normal. But then . . . they weren't.

●　●　●　●　●

"I was married to a wonderful slave, and we have two boys," my Sadistic Bastard Patrick wrote me. "My ex-slave took to the Lifestyle like a duck to water. I would not have married her if she hadn't." She addressed Patrick as "Master" in front of the boys when they were young, before changing to "Sir" as they got older.

"There are many that are raising children while living the Lifestyle. Some keep the Lifestyle hidden and then there are some that live it right in front of the children and bring up their children within the Lifestyle." His own children were reared around it but were never exposed to the sex and play.

He then quoted from an email I'd sent him: " 'Maybe I'd make a great submissive because I love you taking control and telling me what I need to know.' "

I wonder if I had really meant that or was just trying to "play" him to get more information. I have no idea.

"I must say I was a bit surprised by it," he wrote.

I was, too. Where had my head been?

But Patrick was surprised because of our phone conversation when I'd said I'd have to be a Dominant because of my lack of trust in anyone. He interpreted my reversal—my submissive comment—as a willingness to be honest and open-minded.

Maybe he was right. I know I certainly wanted to be open-minded. It was my job.

From there, Patrick returned to the topic of trust, the trust a slave must have in a Master to give over control. "The Lifestyle is not all about the large things that control is given over," he said. "It is the small things as well, and in most cases it is the small things that control is given over that mean the most." From the Dominant's point of view, the Dominant takes great responsibility in His or Her control because He/She knows how easily trust can be broken and how hard it is to rebuild that trust once it is shattered, he said. "As a writer, I am sure you know how difficult it can be to put into words what something is. To put a rose into words can be done, but to know a rose one has to hold it and smell it for themselves.

"With this in mind, there might be some things you can do to help understand some things about this Lifestyle. Now I would in no way suggest you stand in front of someone with a whip in his hand. That would be nuts to say the least. But there are some things on the safer side that might help.

"Remember back to our phone conversation. We talked about trust on a scale of one to ten—one meaning no trust and ten meaning one would jump off the roof if told.

"If you would write down and not having to show it to Me—this is for you—write down on a scale from one to ten the trust you have in Me. If you like, you can go back to our first conversation. Each time the trust goes up or down make a side note of why it moved and how it felt and just keep track of it and try and be as honest as you can.

"Try to keep in mind that a lot of what this Lifestyle is about is being honest with ourselves and dealing with what is in the darkest reaches of our minds. Dealing with ourselves on an open and honest level is not always easy to do."

Once again, I sat silent.

Chapter 8

. . . . .

I sat in the darkness of a 1980s Beverly Hills fern bar with a man on whom I'd once had a crush. Years before he'd walked through my L.A. apartment door and our eyes had locked. "Where's your wife?" I'd said. He and she were supposed to join several of us for dinner.

"We're separated," he'd replied. I'd had no way of knowing. I hadn't seen the man since I was a child and he was a married college student. Back then, he'd entertained me with his humor and zest. Twenty years later, he was forty or more. I was on that cusp between mid and late twenties. I was shy and insecure. He was outgoing and confident. And his eyes twinkled, especially when he looked at me. I fell for him with one look. I wouldn't call what we did after that dating. It was more like lustful hanging out.

On one of those lustful evenings, a friend of his approached me and said, "You seem like a really nice girl. I think you should know . . ." He informed me that my crush wasn't actually separated, he was still fully married. By then I didn't care. I was hooked on him. He, however, was hooked on many. We eventually eased our separate ways.

Still, on very rare occasions, and after his wife divorced him, he and I got together as friends. He was brilliant, had more success than I, more notoriety, and more respect, at least for his acting talent. He also made me laugh. That's why we sat in that Beverly Hills fern bar.

"Are we going to have sex tonight?" he asked.

"Maybe some night, but not tonight," I laughed.

He ordered another round of drinks as the beat of Michael Jackson bounced off the picture window panes and I gazed at the young, handsome, yearning-to-be-an-actor tending bar with a smile and a hard chest. Around us, silk-shirted sons of sheiks tapped out dollars and lines to impress the girls seeking the attention of middle-echelon record executives and actors.

"Are we going to have sex tonight?" my friend asked again. The more he drank, the more he repeated his question, and each time I laughed and recited, "Maybe some night, but not tonight."

We finally left the noise and commotion of that Beverly Hills bar to drive down Wilshire Boulevard to my apartment. We took the elevator up to my one-bedroom home and sat side-by-side on my sky blue sofa. I read him bits of sex scenes from one of my novels. I had dreams of being a *New York Times* best-selling writer who was a cross between Jackie Collins and Larry McMurtry. And I trusted my brilliant friend's opinion.

"Are we going to have sex tonight?" he asked.

Though his persistent query was beginning to get irksome, I laughed again, "Not tonight, but . . ."

He dropped to the floor, on his knees, unzipped his pants, and pulled out his penis. "Do you have a place where I can stick this?"

I gaped at it. "No," I chuckled nervously. It was huge. *No wonder that thing had hurt so.* Years before, I'd given this man my virginity.

I'd like to specifically recall that I gave it to him before I found out he wasn't separated, but I'm not sure. I do remember that we slept together only once, on a December night. Back then, I'd wanted to have sex with him again. Now I didn't, not at all.

"Do you have a place where I can stick this?"

"No," I laughed.

He grabbed my hand and pulled it over to his member. I jerked back my arm, but he was stronger than I. I think I fell toward him, but I'm not certain, because I found myself standing on the other side of the room. Breathing heavily, I stated hard, "I think it's time for you to go."

He stared at me, his eyes wide with disbelief.

"I think it's time for you to go," I repeated.

I watched him through the darkness. The sounds of traffic filtered up the five flights into my apartment as I waited to see if he was going to lunge toward me. Then, I saw a click in his brown eyes as if he came to.

Slowly, he stood, zipped up his pants, and walked out the door, never saying a word. I waited a moment before I followed him, peered out the door and down the hallway. He was about to round the corner to the elevator when I called out, "Are you angry with me?"

I'm not good with people being angry at me. In fact, I'll do most anything to soothe their souls. My mother taught me that. "Anything for peace," she said. "Anything for peace."

My friend glared at me, turned the corner, and left, never saying a word.

I was devastated.

· · · · ·

I never did Patrick's task. Perhaps I was lazy. Perhaps I didn't trust enough. I'd trusted my friend and that hadn't worked out so well. But if I did Patrick's task now, I'd say he was an eight to ten all the way. And the reason for that is that he was always kind and a gentleman. But on a scale of one to ten in importance, I trusted him because he never made one advance toward me. Not even a single innuendo. I appreciated that.

Chapter 9

. . . . .

Roger was a married Vietnam veteran from the Hill Country of central Texas. He contacted me after reading my Alt.com posting. By then, I was so tired of answering men's questions about me without them providing additional information about themselves, or insisting that we meet "eye-to-eye" before communicating more, that I was being cautious with my details.

"I understand your need to keep information about yourself secret until we are better acquainted," he said. "I feel the same way about myself. So where do we go from here? Neither of us wants to reveal much information until a trust has been established."

But the next day Roger emailed me that he was "somewhat satisfied" that I was legit. "I'll call you Suzy and you can call me Coyote. Feel free to ask me anything you want and I will take it one question at a time. . . . Are you okay with that?"

I was, so I simply asked him what brought him to Alt.

"Curiosity about the lifestyle," he answered. "The desire to add excitement and variety to my sex life. A change of pace from my rather humdrum sex life at home."

Over several days and several emails Coyote explained that he and his wife "are the 'Sinner and the Saint.'" She was a godly woman who'd grown up devoutly Catholic and continued that practice into adulthood, making sure their children were in church every Sunday, and going to church twice a week herself. In contrast, Coyote's mother had taken him to church only a few times, primarily on religious holidays. Otherwise, they didn't go. Coyote still doesn't go.

Like Dusty, Coyote had mentioned to his wife that he'd like to try some different things sexually, though unlike Dusty, Coyote hadn't been specific in what he wanted to try.

"But she just says ok, maybe the next time."

He and his wife did have sex—whenever he asked. But he felt she was doing it only out of duty as his wife. So Coyote decided to not mention spicing up their sex life, unless his wife broached the topic first. "Then I will know she is doing it because she wants to, not because I ask her to." And like Dusty, Coyote decided to do what he felt he needed to do to get sexual satisfaction, without his wife's knowledge.

"I love her dearly and would never want to hurt her in any way. She is a wonderful person. We just differ on our sexual desires."

I wrote back with a couple more questions.

The next morning Coyote emailed me asking if I'd be offended if he answered my questions in his "own words and lingo instead of trying to stay proper." I didn't mind. And that night, just as promised, he sat down at his computer and pecked out his answer.

My wife will do oral on me, but I feel like she is not really into it. The rule is absolutely no cumming in her mouth. I love the feeling when I cum in a mouth. I guess it is the suction on my penis while I am cumming. It feels like I cum more than usual and makes me feel totally drained. When I do oral on her, she stiffens up and says it tickles. She tries to act like she enjoys it for my sake, I guess, but I can tell she is not relaxing like I want her to and had rather move on to intercourse, which we usually do. I would prefer more foreplay and having her completely relaxed and ready before we

start the actual intercourse. After we have been having intercourse for 15 or 20 minutes, she says she is getting dry, which she
is, and that tells me she is not truly enjoying it. We stop intercourse. I masturbate until I cum and shoot it on her tits. This is
how about 95% of our lovemaking sessions are. Same ole, same
ole. And anal is out of the question. However, that is ok with me.
I have done it on male and female. I enjoyed it, but I can take it
or leave it. If my partner wants it, then that's what is important
to me—doing it because you like it and are into it.

"I have done it on male and female." Those words reverberated
in my ears as loudly as if I'd heard him speak them rather than read
them. That's because I hadn't expected them from him—a married
Vietnam vet, living in central Texas, who called himself Coyote.

Everything I'd read about bisexuality had indicated that it wasn't
uncommon in young women—in fact, it was downright trendy—but
it was *not* common in men, presumably of any age.

I thought about Richard, my forty-one-year-old navy man. He
was continuing to have sex with men. Even Dusty, my gun-toting,
Vietnam vet/married Texas rancher would soon email me that he
longed to have sex with a man, under a woman's direction and
involvement. Eventually, a retired army man/married high school
principal would contact me confessing that he, too, was searching
for a man with whom to have sex. Like Dusty, as well as Richard,
he'd prefer a woman to be involved.

· · · · ·

Coyote said he had a "normal family life" until he was fourteen or
fifteen years old, when what he described as his father's "drinking
problem" escalated and eventually both of his parents cheated. His
parents divorced, remarried each other, and divorced again.

"I'm not sure if my childhood affected my sexual desires or not.
I don't feel like it did, but I really have no way of knowing. I just

know that my desires started early in life. I have always had the attitude that if it feels good and I enjoy it, go for it."

Since Coyote's parents didn't talk to him about sex, he got his sex education from his friends, older boys bragging about their sexual accomplishments, and older adults, including a man named "George." George was in his sixties and Coyote was sixteen or seventeen when he and his buddies began spending time with the retired widower.

"He was always letting young guys come to his house and drink a few beers after we got out of school." In return, they drove him to the grocery store and on other errands, since George didn't have a car. But George made sure the boys were always indebted to him. "He would pay us for this or just lend us a few bucks when we asked."

One Saturday night, Coyote and his friends gathered at George's to party. "Most of us decided to stay there overnight. The bedding was limited, so George offered to let me and another guy sleep in his bed with him. He slept in the middle (convenient huh?). I had sensed that he might be queer so I did not object to sleeping in his bed with him since I was horny as always.

"I lay there for a while to see if he would do anything. After it was obvious that the other boy was asleep—or more like passed out—George started tossing and turning some as if he was asleep but restless. Eventually he started putting his hand on my thigh and it finally ended up in my crotch. I was laying there with a throbbing hard-on. Once he felt it, he knew I was awake and ready. He began by stroking me slow and easy. After a few minutes he whispered to me, 'Can I take it?' I said yes and he eased down and started sucking me. He had taken his teeth out before getting in bed. He was very gentle and thorough, and swallowed every drop of my cum. I think to this day that is probably the best blowjob I have ever had. Maybe that is why I keep wanting more, in hopes of matching that first blowjob. And too, the risk of being caught by the other guy waking up seemed to be part of the thrill."

Coyote closed with "Suzy, I want you to know I think this is really weird. Here I am spilling my guts out to someone I don't even know. These are things I have kept locked up for over 35 yrs. and wanting to tell someone. I just never have had the chance to tell anyone I trusted enough. But then again, I don't know you and you don't know me. In a way that makes me feel safe telling you. It feels good.

"Thanks."

After the thanks, Coyote inserted a red rose icon.

His virtual flower and words splashed upon my heart like raindrops refreshing the desert floor. I sat silently at my computer and soaked them in. It felt good to make someone feel safe, to help someone open up and be honest. And it felt *so* nice to be appreciated, to be complimented. I didn't know what I'd do without my sex freaks. They were so good to me.

Chapter 10

. . . . .

But my job was to listen and report, not listen and help. As my shrink—the woman I was seeing to help me with relationships—would tell me, I wasn't anyone's therapist. Nor were my sex freaks my therapist . . . or my friends. They were my sources. I reminded myself I was—I am—a journalist.

And I was a journalist with a dearth of female sex sources. Women weren't responding to my AFF and Alt postings, so I returned to Craigslist and posted in the strictly platonic section in Providence, Rhode Island. "I'm looking for some great women who will let me delve into their sex lives for a book I'm writing about sex." With that one posting, I got a response that had me immediately hitting the keyboard: "I am 23, female, and a virgin."

I didn't know that twenty-three-year-old virgins still existed. Holly was not only a virgin, but a recent college graduate who'd just moved to Providence from the Pacific Northwest. "Can you tell me your definition of being a virgin?" I asked. "And why you decided to maintain your virginity?"

"My definition of virginity is loose, excuse the pun," she replied. "I would say that sex encompasses all forms of intimacy right down to heavy petting, dry humping, oral, etc. But to be technical, virginity is a claim made by someone who has never experienced vaginal penetration. With the exception of penetration, I have experienced all other forms of sexual activity. I suppose a 'true' virgin is one who has never experienced any form of sex. However, I feel it fair to say that while a kiss is part of sex, it is not sex. Therefore where do we draw the line? That is why I feel virginity, in its crudest form, is simply without penetration."

That made sense to me.

"I have a lengthy history as to why I am a virgin. To start, I will tell you I was raised in a fundamental church unknown by most. They are a very private Christian sect that seeks to exclude themselves from all worldly life. They are very good people, are nonjudgmental or rather no more so than most I know, and I still hold them in the highest regard. While I am not affiliated with them any longer, my life still retains much of their doctrine, virginity included."

• • • • •

Non-judgmental. I repeated the word in my head. *Non-judgmental.* The opposite of judgmental. "Do not judge lest you be judged yourselves," Jesus said.

That summer I'd been in Eugene, Oregon, and stared at the black-light poster of sexual positions inspired by the *Kama Sutra*, the members of my church youth choir and I had spent our days going door-to-door talking to people about Jesus and inviting them to our concerts of contemporary Christian music. We'd spent our nights singing our Christian songs to shopping mall crowds, my toes happily tapping in my white leather Bernardo sandals. And I'd spent my very late nights huddled in a darkened dormitory room listening to a friend, for whom I cared deeply, express her guilt over sleeping with her boyfriend. She rationalized their intercourse by saying they were in love, that one day they'd marry, and so they were fulfilling God's rule that a man leave his mother and father to cleave to his wife. Thus, she and her boyfriend were no longer two individuals; they were one, just as Jesus had directed in Matthew 19:4–6.

My fellow teenager quoted those three Bible verses to support her point of view. They were the very same verses I pointed to solid as stone in my belief that premarital sex was a sin and the very reason I worried about my friend and her heart and soul. I may have been a good listener then, but I certainly was not one without judgment. And I most definitely didn't think about the fact that the Ten Commandments, like my beliefs, had been written in stone. And that stone had been broken, just like I would break my own beliefs about the time that Holly had been born.

"For in the same way you judge, you will be judged," Jesus said. "And by your standard of measure, it shall be measured to you."

I desperately yearned to be non-judgmental with my sex freaks. It was my job. And it is my faith.

· · · · ·

"Like most young girls," Holly said, "I fell in love for the first time and was deeply hurt afterwards." He was a young man from her church who she believed was more committed to their faith than she. "In all honesty, I would have lost my virginity to him if he would have allowed it. At that point in my life, I began to fathom how much of a role sex played in my life. I now realize I am an extremely sexual person, a conundrum since I don't have sex."

Holly now felt "stuck" with what is "supposed to be" her "most sacred possession"—her virginity.

"I am old enough to know better than to have sex with the first person I encounter," she said. "However, I am now in a place where I don't feel the need to wait until marriage like I was raised to believe. Hence, I am unable to allow sex as a viable option until I fall in love again. . . . Most are waylaid by this and exclaim at what I am missing. But I ask, 'How do I miss it, if I've never had it?'"

Holly had me nodding, this time in understanding.

"Presently, I still consider myself a Christian, but not in a tradi-tional sense of the term," she wrote. "I do not take the Bible at face value. I do not feel there are any black and white issues or that everything in the Bible is correctly interpreted."

. . . . .

I took the Bible literally, when I was at Baylor. In fact, when one of my religion professors suggested that the visions in the Old Testa-ment were drug-induced, I was appalled, outraged, dumbstruck. I found the very idea to be blasphemous and an insult to Yahweh. There was no way this professor could be a Christian, I believed, and I wondered why in the world he was allowed to teach at Baylor. (Maybe that's why I received a D in his class.)

Years later, as I covered press conferences, my black-and-white beliefs began to gray. Repeatedly, I was amazed at how a group of reporters could attend the same event, hear the exact same words, and leave with such differing interpretations of those words. One reporter would write that speaker X said Y, while another reporter would write speaker X didn't say Y, he said Z.

That's when I realized that though the Bible is inspired by God, it is written by fallible human beings. And while Jesus may have said and meant X, Matthew may have heard Y, while John heard Z.

Maybe God intended it to be that way. Maybe He wants His message to uniquely apply to each individual's heart and needs.

. . . . .

With Holly's move to Rhode Island, she started to date, her attempt "to end a dry spell." She then noted that her mother had "ALWAYS" dated in between her four husbands.

Four husbands. I read those two words as many times as I had the word "non-judgmental."

I also believed that this bit of information was significant—that her mother's marital history, beauty, and "uncanny charm," as

Holly described it, had probably affected Holly's self-esteem and outlook on love, life, marriage, and sex. Perhaps they had affected her even more than the non-judgmental fundamentalist sect that she had been so willing to discuss. But Holly streaked by this mother-dating-divorce data as if it were a mere acquaintance to whom she was willing to give only a passing nod of hello.

"I am anticipating without joy when I must explain my virginity." But she knew that wouldn't be that difficult to do. "I find most men enjoy on some level the fact [that] I am a virgin. It feeds their fantasies on some level, especially since I don't have qualms with other intimacies. Of course every man I've been with feels they are sure to be the one who will help ease my transition into being sexually active."

Still, Holly sometimes wondered if she'd ever have sex. "As I get older, I get farther from the young girl in high school who thought she was going to hell for letting a boy feel her up over her shirt. I do not feel remorse, which scares me now. . . . I moved away to start over, to not let myself get trapped by religion, marriage, to force myself to create a life from scratch.

"After I moved, I had an epiphany of sorts. I thought, 'I can have sex!' It frightens me to meet the person I will be afterwards. Will I be without? Is my virginity so inherent in what makes up my person that I will be lacking? I think sometimes my sexual frustrations make life interesting. Then I wonder if I am avoiding sex for the sake of keeping it interesting. I think, though, after experiencing sex, a new dimension will open up. There will be a new fold in the fabric of my life."

I was silent as I read her words . . . and read them over and over. They rolled in my head like the clanking rush of letters in a bingo cage. And they wouldn't stop. . . .

Chapter 11

. . . . .

Who would I be after I finished this book?

And perhaps more importantly, or more worrisome, would my family accept me afterward?

Once, in the darkness of a New Year's Eve party, I joked that my mother didn't think I'd ever kissed anyone. No one believed me until the hostess, who knew my mother very, very well, said, "Oh, yes, she's telling the truth." I think I was in my thirties at the time.

So if my mother didn't think I'd ever kissed a man when I was in my thirties, how would she look at me when she discovers that I am no longer a virgin?

She—no, my entire family—is of the don't even think it, don't tell it belief. And here I am thinking and telling—thinking and telling more than I ever intended.

How can you embarrass me like this?

I hear her decades-old words. And in my mind, I argue with her: Because if I'm going to ask my sex freaks to be honest, then I have to be equally honest.

No, you don't. You're the reporter. Not the source.

But . . . but . . . the truth will set you free. Isn't that what I was taught in church? The truth will set you free.

The preacher, your Sunday school teacher, the Bible—they weren't talking about that kind of truth. They were talking about the truth of Jesus.

And my head sinks into my hands.

Why is a fifty-year-old woman obsessed with what she imagines her eighty-year-old mother thinks?

It's that dead daddy thing.

I've run across it so many times in my life when I've met people whose father died when they were kids, especially if that child was the youngest—we feel responsible for the safety and happiness of our mothers.

I remember the exact moment that happened for me. I was five years old. I was standing in the living room of our house, peering down the long hallway to the master bedroom. My mother sat on the floor of the bedroom, the black telephone to her ear, crying. Weeping over my dead daddy. I knew at that very moment that I was never going to hurt her like that. I was never going to make her cry like that. I would protect her. I would take care of her.

If I had walked down that hallway and stood behind her and watched her back shake as she wept, in my memory, I would have been tall enough to reach down to her, because in my mind, at five years old, I was the height I am now—five feet, seven inches. And she was child size when she was slumped in tears.

Forty-five years after I watched my mother cry, I still don't want to make her weep. I don't want to upset her. I don't want to disappoint her. She's had enough of that.

Holly had what she called a "burden." I had what I called a "secret." And through this book, I was revealing that secret—a secret that would devastate my mother.

Yes, Holly was right.

No matter whether it happens with a true love, an infatuation, a crush, a friend, an acquaintance, a stranger, a molester, or a rapist, the loss of one's virginity changes a person forever. Perhaps it is the one event that is as significant as being born. It affects one's very being—the soul, the essence. One is no longer who one once was.

I could get up and leave my desk, blank out my mind, or fill my brain with something other than thoughts of Holly and our shared virginity identity fears. I did all three. I got up and left my desk. I grabbed my eighteen-pack of oatmeal raisin cookies and a sixteen-ounce glass of nonfat milk and ate six 120-calorie cookies and drank two 180-calorie glasses of milk. The 1080 calories filled my brain and blocked the pain. I went back to my desk and computer and clicked open the next email.

Chapter 12

• • • • •

"please. i do enjoy talking about sex and my sex life a great deal so if i can be of any assistance, i would be more than happy to oblige."

"More than happy to oblige"—I liked that. It sounded sincere. Her name was Jessica. She was twenty-five years old and had grown up in greater Chicago, the upper middle class product of a Jewish mother and Catholic father, rendering her, as she said, "Jewish by default."

"i am openly bisexual, though i have been struggling either way for years, since i was 19."

She also typed only in lowercase, declaring that capital letters slowed her down.

"actually, i don't know if struggle is the right word. just trying to figure it all out. i still feel like i'm just sitting on the fence, trying to decide one way or the other, and i don't want to."

When Jessica was eleven years old, she discovered her parents' copy of *The Joy of Sex*. It got her, she said, "very excited, but not in a way i could translate into action." Like seemingly everyone I talked to—no matter their generation—her parents didn't talk to her about sex. "i guess the assumption was that i wasn't even leaning in that direction so they were safe." Also, Jessica was expected to be good and self-sufficient as her parents' focus was on her disabled younger brother. But at age thirteen, when she began to develop breasts, started menstruating, and got contact lenses, things changed.

She invited her friend Shelby and two boys over and "for some UNKNOWN reason" her parents left them alone in the house. "well, one thing led to another and soon we were playing strip poker and before i knew it we were all up in my parents' bed, shirts off, kissing and rubbing up against each other. then shelby and i would switch boys."

Within a week, almost everyone at Jessica's middle school knew her sex news. "i had such a good girl reputation for so long—now guys were definitely thinking twice about my prudishness and my spot at the lunch table moved on towards the top. i liked that. i loved it, actually."

A month later, she, Shelby, and another girl friend were with thirteen boys, who taunted Jessica about her sexual exploits, claiming she'd performed oral sex. Their taunts, along with goading, worked. After asking if she could get pregnant from a blowjob and being assured she couldn't, Jessica lay down on her back. A boy straddled her chest. "and we were off and running." Once again, the girls took turns with the boys.

The next day, when even more girls in "the upper echelons" of her lunch table performed oral sex on more boys so that they "could all be on the same base," Jessica became known as "The Motivator." She was "simultaneously elated and petrified."

But then the school principal and Jessica's mother heard her sex gossip. She denied the facts to them both. To her thirty friends who phoned, she "meekly" confessed. Her mother berated her, "Do you know what this could do to our reputation in the community?"

"i was 13," Jessica wrote me. "i didn't give a rat's ass about my parents' reputation when my name was suddenly being written in bathroom stalls with my number (for a good time call jessica . . .) and desks were etched with the same information."

There were unwanted repercussions, though. One of the boys on whom she'd performed oral sex frequently blocked her path in the school hallway, pressed his groin against her, and jeered, "You know where you want it," while his crew of gaping-mouthed, giggling thirteen-year-old males watched.

Jessica then noted to me, "every year, on the day, i will remember and think back, not in any sort of, wow, wasn't that an amazing day? but more so in a wow, this day x number of years ago really changed my life."

· · · · ·

Jessica captivated me. We were so different. When I was in high school in the very early 1970s, I'm not sure I knew there was such a thing as oral sex, though I heard there was lots of making out going on in the church steeple. And in very stark contrast to Jessica, when I got home from school each day, I grabbed a two-pack of Hostess chocolate cupcakes and a glass of milk, lay down on the couch by myself, and watched reruns of *I Love Lucy*, where Lucy and Ricky slept in separate twin beds.

Jessica followed oral sex on a boy with a couple of crushes on girls at summer camp. I spent well more than a decade of summers at camp, and never once did having a crush on a girl occur to me. I'm not sure I knew that girls could like girls. It was beyond my Lucy and Ethel comprehension. Obviously not Jessica's, especially when it came to a camper named Lauren.

"i was very aware of how i touched her because who knew, i was just so aware. that was my first conscious thoughts of something bigger than boys."

She assumed everyone thought about girls the way she did, just no one talked about it. Then, one day she was driving around with her friend Ashley, talking to her about Lauren. "i was describing to ashley how i felt, how it was so nice to be around lauren and how amazing i thought she was. i turned to ashley and said, 'have you ever felt that way about a girl?' 'no, never' she replied, and i almost drove my car off the road. that changed everything."

I presumed Jessica meant it changed everything because she was shocked to learn that not all girls loved girls and that she was embarrassed or ashamed about having such feelings.

No.

"it was the first time i realized that perhaps these feelings didn't come out of nowhere and that they were valid. it was exciting. it made me feel different. it never felt wrong or bad. it was really a revelation that i was happy to have had. of course, i kept it mainly to myself as i didn't want to freak anyone out and really, i had to wrap my own brain around it."

While she wrapped her brain around it, Jessica, then a high school senior, focused on a sophomore boy. Two months after they started dating, they decided to have intercourse.

"we started making out and once he had an erection, i slipped the condom on and presto, chango, JESUS CHRIST, did it hurt or what? it did, but we carried on until he came. i did not."

In the four years they were intimate, she never had an orgasm with him and never told him she didn't.

"i would occasionally, when he gave good head or we had sex for a long time, get something called orgasmic paralysis, when my breathing patterns would change and i would feel tingly all over my body—shortness of breath, i imagine."

Jessica's senior year in high school culminated with pornography and handcuff play.

Mine culminated with maybe one date—if I had one, I don't remember it—and the most boring graduation ever not recorded. If I had sat on the back porch doing decoupage by myself, it would have been more exciting.

I had to move on.

But the more I talked with people about their sex lives, the more a strange thing began to happen to me—I began losing what little sex drive I'd ever had. Siouxsie Ramone—a sweet, punked out, chain-smoking, twenty-five-year-old phone sex operator who had been molested several times when she was five, who had had sex more than once with a teenager who had forced her into intercourse when she had no comprehension of what they were doing (she was twelve), and who had been beaten by boyfriends when she was a teenager, despite the fact that her mother saw the bruises on her child's body (and didn't intervene)—suggested that I was losing my desire for sex because I was hearing "all the bad side."

Maybe.

She also told me—as we chatted on the phone—that she had quit her phone sex job after a man asked her to role-play a seven-year-old girl.

We were both silent after that . . . until she broke the quiet. "And I was just like, uh, yeah, no—because if he's calling and doing that, then who's to say that he's not doing that in his home life."

Or maybe my desire was dying because I always seemed to find something in these people's lives to which I could connect. Siouxsie's father had died when she was three months old.

"I look like him," she said.

I look like my father, too.

I had to move on again. My soul was feeling Siouxsie's soul, and when it did, I had to sit in quiet pain. I didn't want to do that. I reached for another oatmeal cookie and returned to Jessica.

Maybe it was because there was something about Jessica that made me feel like she was in control of her sex life rather than it being in control of her; maybe it was because I never talked with Jessica on the phone and never heard her voice so that it could linger in my ears long after we'd hung up; or maybe it was because I had nothing in common with her. All I know is that my communication with Jessica was easier on me emotionally.

Her sophomore year in college, she moved into a co-op, which she described as a "breeding ground for sex." She had a new boyfriend, and he, as well as Lauren, the girl Jessica had wanted for three years, and Lauren's boyfriend were at a party at the co-op. But Jessica didn't give a hoot that her own boyfriend was there because she "got hammered," to use her terminology, and, via a kissing game, she and Lauren kissed. And they kissed again. "and it was so soft, so good."

Meanwhile, two other women were trying to get together a five-girl orgy, so Jessica went up to their floor. There, she ran into Lauren and her boyfriend, "who had been plotting. i don't know what words were said but before i knew it, i was willingly pushed into my bedroom and was going at it full force with lauren while her boyfriend watched and chain-smoked.

"huge. momentous. i was going down on a woman i had lusted after for YEARS. i could hardly stand it. . . . she went down on me, la la la. it was just so nice, it was so nice, so so nice. goodness. i had my bout of orgasmic paralysis and was so excited."

Jessica phoned all of her friends to tell them about it and, subsequently, considered herself bisexual. She believed she was bisexual until she was twenty-one years old, when she moved to San Francisco and had a three-year relationship with a woman.

"i was so so so into her, would've died for her at some point i swear, that i didn't think she would ever be into me if she thought i was anything less than gay, even though when i first met her she knew that i was bi and it was never a problem. so i made a decision. i came out to my family (they were fine with it, not terribly surprised), cut off my hair, and changed my wardrobe."

I was stunned. My mother would have yelled, "No! You're not a lesbian!"

"all of my good friends supported me but with some trepidation—they knew me well enough to not entirely buy it. but i did. i really wanted to be gay. i really wanted to just be done with the fence-sitting and the back and forth. and so many bisexual girls are not really bisexual. they sleep with men, men, men and then once in a blue moon sleep with women. and pure, die-hard lesbians have never been supportive of women who sleep with both. i hated that stereo-type, hated the boxed in feel of it. being a lesbian was so cool, so new. there was a whole new scene, a whole new lingo. i loved it—for two and half years. then i cheated on my girlfriend with a dude and came back to the fence."

The reason was simple: "i always stay more interested when i don't really know where i stand and the other person seems to wield more power. after those two years, the playing fields leveled, and i started to lose interest. the sex, which had been fantastic (dildo and strap-ons and what not) and these lesbians i had been so keen on knowing or getting to know became people and lost their allure."

. . . . .

When Jessica and I first met through Craigslist, she'd only recently ended her San Francisco lesbian relationship and moved to Atlanta, where she was working as a chef in one of the city's finest hotels. In the South, Jessica took on the appearance of a typical, straight college student, which made her look much younger than her twenty-five years, and started looking for male lovers.

"as i get older, i've learned what it takes for me to have an orgasm," she said. "i could always masturbate myself to one but somehow when i was with another person i couldn't translate (and was very shy) about trying to explain what it would take. in the past two years, i have learned to get involved in the process and not be ashamed or embarrassed about it. . . . i always hear about women in their seventies who finally have an orgasm (with or without part-ner) and i am happy to have reached a point with myself where i can ask for what i need. being able to communicate, that's what makes it great. and asking for what i want. i'm getting very good at that.

"the physical fulfillment is fantastic and when it comes with emotional intimacy, even better. but i realized, towards the end of my last relationship, that all the emotional connection in the world was not saving our sex life. i believe they have to exist in tandem,

but right now, i would much rather have a fantastic physical connection and a less strong emotional one than vice versa. i don't want
to sacrifice sex for long, involved conversations. i feel there will be
plenty of time for that later on in life. that's why i have friends."

Oh, gosh, I understood.

To me, love and sex are two very different entities.

To me, there is no balance, no happy medium, no in-between
between friendship without sex and an obsessive, controlling relationship with sex. Besides, I know that no matter what, a man is
going to eventually leave you by death or divorce, so why bother?
At least that's what I've observed from childhood to adulthood.

Chapter 13

· · · · ·

J.D. was a married Texan who contacted me through AdultFriend-Finder. According to his AFF profile, he "left no pussy uneaten." According to my profile of him, he didn't type apostrophes. "Hey, girl, lets talk," he opened.

"If you're interested in talking only, that's cool," I replied. "But if you're looking for sex, that wouldn't be journalistically ethical for me to do."

J.D., who claimed to have a "long, thick" endowment, was still game for us to talk. He gave me his private email address and said, "Lets see what happens."

I ignored his "lets see what happens" and dove into a list of questions, culminating with a plea I now regret: "Educate me about the world of the Internet and sex, please . . . as well as about yourself." It was that plea part that I regretted. *Please.* It sounded so desperate, so childish, so unprofessional. But at least it worked. It kept our communication going.

"I decided to use the internet to find women because being married doesn't give me any time to cruise the bars like I did when I was younger. I'm 57 now, and AFF gives me access to married women who are as frustrated as I am. It also cuts through the shit of trying to date while married, no need to lie and try to keep up with them to every woman I date. Right now it is paying off at about a 10 percent ratio to emails sent. . . ."

Ten years into his current marriage, which is his second, J.D. decided to start cheating. His wife had gone through menopause, after which, according to J.D., "she didnt want sex at all, no way, no how. I went along with it, no sex, for 4 years, then decided to do this. I refuse to do without sex ever again. Prostitutes are out of the question, too many things can go wrong. . . . And porn sites just dont hold any interest to me. I guess more than sex, its just the closeness I miss most."

That line stopped me. *It's just the closeness I miss most.*

"The thing I have found out about internet sex is how many people are frustrated like me. As far as your ethics go, I believe Dr. Kinsey dabbled in his research so he would know first hand about what he was trying to figure out about sex."

With that reference to Dr. Alfred Kinsey and the *Kinsey Report*, studies on human sexual behavior done in the 1940s and 1950s, I knew my plea had been misinterpreted, just as I should have known it would have been. On top of that, I still couldn't believe how many men came on to me without knowing a thing about me or what I looked like.

According to J.D.'s self-description—besides being well-endowed—he was six feet, four inches tall and a bit on the plump side. He'd gone to college but hadn't finished. He was self-employed and a smoker. I guess I should have told J.D. that I don't "do" smokers. But there was a part of me that smiled at the way J.D. spoke to me.

"Dear Heart,"—I almost stopped and grabbed my heart at that—"the majority of my experiences have been good, but, as in life, you dont always hit it off with everyone. The worst part about it is that every woman on here gets spoiled by all the emails they get, they forget that a one-eyed crack whore will get as many answers as they are getting, and get the attitude that they are the hottest thing online."

So much for my ego-boosting.

"The majority of them forget that AFF is an adult site, and they still ask for walks in the moonlight or on the beach, not going to happen, unless they want to fuck on the beach."

With that, I noticed that J.D. also leaned toward the use of commas when he should have used periods. I guess flirtation can make me forget punctuation, and a slap of reality makes me notice it.

"My best meet was a married nurse, we still see each other 1 or 2 days a week, and are going to put an ad in as a couple to meet more people. The majority of the women who will actually meet are overweight, older married women who don't get any at home, and their egos need building up."

Oh, shit. I felt like he *was* describing me.

"Some are very nice and weight is not an issue with me, so its a win, win situation. The worst that happened so far is the guys who write pretending to be girls, but you can read between the lines and weed them out. So, dear, whats your favorite fetish? Sometimes they are not so strange when you say them out loud."

Something flitted through my brain as I read J.D.'s fetish question, but I wouldn't allow it to slow down enough to let me to know what it was. Yet I found myself mentally grinning that "they are not so strange when you say them out loud." Still, I ignored his question to me. "Tell me about the guys writing and pretending to be girls and how you weed them out," I said.

"Dear heart, the way I weed out men is to read the ads, if the guy says hes bi-curious, thats a sign, if, when you correspond with them the wife is always out of town, or he wants to meet you for drinks without her, an abnormal interest in the size and girth of my dick, so he can tell the wife, and the biggest hint is when he wants to know if I have a lot of body hair, lots of bear lovers out there."

"Bear lovers"—J.D. was referring to men who love hairy men.

To use J.D.'s phrasing again, he had been "heavy" into the swing lifestyle for twelve years between his first and second marriages. "A swingers club is about the only place to go if you want to be wild without worrying about the old blowjob under the table, no worry about going to jail or offending anyone."

He and his nurse girlfriend currently were looking for couples, primarily. "She likes to eat pussy, but a dick is still needed." If a second penis wasn't included, she got upset that J.D. was getting more sex than she. That didn't stop J.D. from adding the kicker: "Would be willing to meet you in Houston for drinks, both of us, and SHOW you how we like to fuck."

In what seemed to be becoming my modus operandi, I ignored his offer. "I love wells of info. How did you get into the lifestyle? And since you weren't married, who did you take since guys without girls aren't invited?" I knew that most swing clubs didn't allow single men. "Tell me more. Tell me anything/everything."

At the time, I simply was trying to keep our communication going. But in retrospect, I wonder if my shrink would have considered that flirtation.

"Suzy dear," he responded.

I have to admit that I still love the way he addressed me.

"I always took my current girlfriend at the time, and several clubs would allow single men, for a steep cover charge. Some couples would prefer to fuck with just an extra guy for the little lady, usually older guys who couldn't get it up anymore. At least you didn't have to worry about them butt fucking you. I got into this because I have always been very sexual in nature, I guess because a neighbor woman gave me some pussy when I just turned 11, and I've been enthralled by women ever since."

My gosh, he was using apostrophes. And, oh, yeah, if J.D. was telling me the truth, he'd been sexually abused as a child and apparently didn't consider it abuse—par for the course.

"Also, like most men, I'm very visual in nature, and with all the nudity at a swingers club, it suits my needs. That's why I go to the nudist camp in Navasota [Texas] pretty regular. Its now for adults only and they have a dance every Sat night, which fills all my needs. Maybe I could take you. Are you that interested in your research? You can answer my questions, Suzy. I don't bite; just think we could talk a lot more with some kind of dialog going on. I never have been a long-winded guy."

* * * * *

Rather than confess to J.D., I emailed a couple of friends of mine, "I'm thinking about sex way too much."

By then, my emails to my buddies had become my daily journal and coping mechanism.

"Today when I was driving downtown, there was an ad on the radio that said come have a margarita on our award-winning deck. I heard come have a margarita on our award-winning dick.

"So . . . I need your advice." I told them about J.D. and his offers to me. "I'm tempted," I admitted. I didn't admit that I was tempted because I wanted to watch real people have sex—not a silicone- or saline-filled, lip-injected, head-to-toe makeup-covered "Barbie" have scripted and directed porn movie sex.

And the reason I wanted to watch real people have real sex was so I could learn how to have sex myself. If there's one thing I know for a fact, it's that I'm very bad at sex—I have no idea what I'm doing. Maybe, just maybe, since this was business for me, I could interview these people and ask them how do you do this and how do you do that.

Stop, Suzy! Think!

I typed to my friends, "But I don't know this guy . . . and there's the safety issue. . . ."

* * * * *

The next day, I emailed J.D.. "You've got to email me the details of when you were 11.

"I do want to do an in-person interview with you and your friend, and I do want to hear about the nudist camp, but I've got to get a bunch of stuff written before I can run over to Houston." At least that was the cop-out excuse I gave him. The truth was that despite the fact that two months had passed since I'd done my one and only face-to-face interview with Frank, the swing club owner, I still hadn't been able to muster the guts to do another in-person interview. It was so much easier to hide in my computer. To listen to others live their lives rather than live a life of my own.

Okay, confession. What had flitted through my mind when J.D. asked me about my fetishes was a memory of a guy I'd briefly dated when I lived in L.A., though I'm not sure "dated" is the right word for what we did. Occasionally, he'd call, I'd go over to his place, and we'd sit on the floor of his dimly lit living room, drink, talk, and he'd show off his latest purchases—clothes, a down comforter, whatever. My job was to ooh and ah. Once or twice we played at intimacy. One time, he asked me what my fantasies were.

"I don't have any," I said.

"I'll come up with one for you."

The fantasy he created was me lying nude on a king-sized bed in a hotel room. I pictured it in Palm Springs, with me surrounded by work, newspapers, and a tray full of room service leftovers, while Headline News played on the TV, back in the days when HLN was called Headline News. My friend pictured himself walking through the door; I look up, and he and his tongue dive into my privates and stay there all night.

I went along with his idea—he looked like Sting. Well, Sting in the 1980s. By "went along," I don't mean we fulfilled it. I'm not sure I ever saw him again after that night. But for years, while traveling on business, as I lay alone in my hotel bed, I saw that scenario in my mind.

Despite J.D.'s query about me, he never had a chance to learn any of my fantasies or fetishes. He never responded to my last email. Then again, what was there to learn about me? Someone else had had to make up a fantasy for me. And I couldn't even remotely comprehend the concept of having *any* fetishes . . . other than a fetish for perfect teeth, which I definitely have.

But regarding J.D., I truly did want to know about his sexual experiences as an eleven-year-old because I wanted to know—to understand—why "my" sex freaks were the way they were.

I thought about Richard . . . and Frank . . . Mr. Golfer . . . Dusty . . . Coyote . . . and so many other men with whom I'd communicated, including Brian, a Vietnam vet, Special Forces. Brian wanted to meet a transsexual or transvestite. "Could I kiss such a person?" he said. "I don't know."

What he did know was that he and his wife of thirty-seven years were sexually disconnected.

> It seems when children come, the spark leaves and there are always so many distractions. I remember we initially slept nude, but that went away. "The kids might see us." What went away was closeness and the tenderness of touch. There were all the competing interests, for me the job. . . . For her, her job and the weight of a mother, volunteer, and a wife. In the pecking order something goes first and something goes last on both sides. So after a while you get tired of rejection. You still long for the tenderness, but it isn't there. Slowly you grow closer in non-physical ways, but the sexuality and satisfaction leave. Oh, when it's discussed, it spurts up, but that too wanes and is gone. If there is a need you either stuff it, turn to self-gratification, or explore the outside. The option to leave the situation is there, but non-physical love, the kids, the family, and the community keep you in.

Brian and I stayed in erratic touch for perhaps a year. As far as I know, he never acted on his fantasies. But his loneliness haunted me. It still does . . . because loneliness seemed to be the universal theme of Americans and their sex lives. More specifically, when it came to married people, particularly men, their loneliness was usually wrapped in a need—not simply a desire—to have someone who would listen without judgment to their most secret sexual desires, whether acted on or not, and accept them, kinks and all.

"Sometimes, my research makes me want to cry," I wrote a friend. "There are so many hurting, lonely, tortured people out there. Sometimes, it makes me laugh. Sometimes, it makes me angry, particularly at men. It's easy for them to hide any humanity when they communicate behind the safety of a computer."

But as time passed, I could block out the thoughts and memories of those men. The people that lingered were the lonesome whippoorwills, their sad songs piercing the midnight darkness like the call of a distant train. They were my Hank Williamses.

Chapter 14

• • • • •

"Look for the table with the chains on it," Albert had said.

Albert was a fifty-year-old, college-educated, Catholic, father, soccer coach, and Bostonian transplanted to Texas. He'd contacted me through Alt.com, where his profile stated he was one-half of a male/female couple looking for submissive couples or women to join in their activities. He claimed to have an average body and be a light/social drinker. His submissive was eight years younger, bisexual, a 36C, with medium-length brown hair, green eyes, and wore contact lenses.

But as Al and I moved from email to phone, I forgot about his partner because he never mentioned her. He talked about bestiality, maintaining that it's more accepted now than in the past and that 1 percent of kinky people practice it. He wouldn't do it, he said, but he'd watch it, as well as anything else. In fact, he once had watched a woman participate in bestiality. "It was beautiful to see her."

From bestiality, his conversation moved to his daughter. I'm not sure I realized then what a jarring transition that was—bestiality to his daughter. For one thing, I think I'd gotten desensitized to the mention of bestiality. Al was at least the third person who'd brought it up. For another, I was too focused on my note-taking. I scribbled that his daughter was assertive, the captain of her soccer team, and he expected she'd be a Domme, a female Dominant, in twenty years.

He also mentioned two very young women he'd taken to The Sanctuary dungeon in Dallas. The ladies had wanted to observe *only*. At first, they were shocked and shaken by what they saw. Two hours later, they were pleading, "Beat me, please, Sir!" he said.

Al offered to escort me to The Sanctuary. I insinuated I might consider it, but I definitely would not be screaming, "Beat me, please, Sir,"—I truly would be going to just watch.

"It can get scary," he said and admitted he'd been a bit frightened the first time he'd attended a public BDSM event, even though the domination, which had occurred in front of forty people, had been more emotional than physical. Al then stated, "If people groping bothers you . . ."

I wasn't about to confess to Al that I hate touch, because right then he told me that he feels evil. And he seemed to revel in his evilness, despite the fact that he also said he believed his role as a Dominant was chivalrous and that he had a "gift" for feeling submissive. Indeed, Al trained as a submissive for eight months to learn how one thinks and feels. The Domme who trained him asked Al if he'd take a bullet for his own submissive.

"Why would I do that?" Al returned.

"Because of what the sub does for you," the Domme answered.

In our second phone conversation, Al warned me, repeatedly, that if my gut ever had qualms about anyone I met on the Internet that I should listen to my gut and run because the Lifestyle is all about truth, honor, honesty, and respect. In fact, that's why Al joined the Lifestyle—truth, honor, honesty, and respect. "No means no." He contended that wasn't always true in the swing world. And that, Al said, was because in the world of swing, only one's sex life was in the other's hand. In BDSM, one's life was in the other's hands.

Those words never left my brain.

And I didn't want to look for the table with chains on it.

But two and a half months had passed since my Valentine's Day interview with Frank. It was past time to stop hiding behind the Internet and time to gut up and get into the real world of alternative sex. In my mind, since I'd done swinging—well, "done" in the sense of sitting outside a bookstore and talking about it with an actual swinger—BDSM was the logical next in-person task. So when Al invited me to a BDSM event—a "munch" at a sports bar, better known in the vanilla world as happy hour—I knew I had to accept. Besides, the munch was just going to be drinks and conversation, not straitjackets and blindfolds, bullwhips and masks. At least I hoped not.

· · · · ·

So on a warm, sunny Wednesday in late April, I find myself reluctantly standing at the edge of the Warehouse District, an area of downtown Austin where thirty-somethings to fifty-somethings meet to drink and find sex. I stare up at the rooftop deck of the two-story Fox and Hound Smokehouse & Tavern. Al had told me the group would be either on the roof of the Fox and Hound or in the tavern's second-floor bar.

Albert also had told me to phone him when I arrived, so that we could find each other easily. I think about the advice Sadistic Bastard had given me seven weeks before: don't ever give out your phone number and always block your number before dialing. Albert had given me the same advice. I phone him. He doesn't answer. I leave a message and walk into the bar.

In the dimness of the room, I don't see a single table with chains on it. I stride through the putrid odor of cigarettes, the eerie glow of countless TVs, the din of bad bar music, and up the stairs. As soon as I hit the second floor, model-pretty waitresses ask if I'm meeting a group.

"Yeah, I'm looking for the table with chains on it."

The ladies look horrified. I turn away. I'm not sure if I spoke those words to intentionally shock or out of guilty confession. I glance up the stairs leading to the rooftop deck. It's closed. But I notice that the stairwell is narrow and poorly lighted—the perfect place for a rape. I notice things like that when I'm alone. I turn back around and spill to the young waitresses that I'm looking for a BDSM group. Maybe my words are begging for protection.

A stunning brunette asks me what BDSM means.

"Bondage, domination, submission, and masochism."

Her mouth drops open. She stares at me. I'm wearing librarian red glasses, a Ralph Lauren sailor blue and white striped T-shirt, and Levi's, just like always. Soccer mom Sesto Meucci slides cover my feet. She walks away in silence. I think I like her shock.

I sit down at the bar, order a Diet Coke, and watch University of Texas softball on the only TV airing women's sports.

Al phones, thank God. Thank God because I don't like sitting here alone.

"Is your friend there?" he asks.

I'd invited a friend along for protection. I try to laugh off that she copped out on me.

He seems pleased. His pleasure twists my nerves.

A waitress leans close and whispers, "There's a table with chains on it downstairs."

I don't budge. I don't want to find the BDSMers by myself.

· · · · ·

Fifteen minutes later, the bulging gut of a fifty-something man in a white button-down shirt with candy-colored stripes comes toward me. I stick out my hand to him—Al had told me what he was wearing. Still, I hadn't expected someone almost as preppy as I. His graying hair is neatly cut and combed. His face is ruddy red as though he spends too much time in the sun and perhaps drinks too much, as well. He reminds me of the stereotypical next-door neighbor—the one to whom you give a friendly wave when you see him grilling burgers and sipping a beer in the backyard.

We walk downstairs to the table with chains. In actuality, there's a lone, silver chain, so small and short that I never would have noticed it. It belongs to Magick, a silent, dark-haired woman in black clothes. Magick's a bit heavy, but firm heavy, just like Al's gut, and proportional. Perfectly applied pink lipstick accentuates her mouth. Black eyeglasses hide her eyes. A heavy, silver-toned, costume jewelry chain loops around her neck.

Al quickly introduces us as he sits down next to her. To Al's right is a young man with a goatee drinking a beer. Next to him is one empty chair. "Is this seat taken?" I say as I start to sit down.

"Yes," Magick answers, her tone relaying that I'm not welcomed.

I grab another stool and inch it in. As soon as I do, Al leaves to get a beer and my spine stiffens—I don't know how to talk to "these people." I sit quietly, feeling awkward in my work. I'm not used to this. I've usually kicked into reporter gear by now.

Al returns and, with beer in hand, proceeds to laugh about a recent BDSM campout. He started drinking at 11 A.M., he says, and they wrapped and bound two nude women, face-to-face, in netting. Then they whipped them.

Too clearly, I see the scene in my head.

Al howls over how much fun it was.

It's not just the image of being bound nude that disturbs me; it's the pain and cruelty of being whipped while naked. Still, I smile, uncomfortably, when, out of the darkness, a man appears. He has a sickly pale pallor. He sits down in the empty chair between Magick and me. Like Magick, he is disconcertingly quiet.

Al suggests we move up to the roof, which has opened.

Magick scoops up her chain from the table and puts it in her purse.

They grab their beers, I grab my Diet Coke, and we troop up two flights of dark, narrow stairs. We sit down at a green metal mesh picnic table, just like the ones at a local insane asylum. I know that because I've written about those tables in one of my true crime books. I want to mention that, in an attempt to contribute *something* to the conversation. But I wonder, too, if I'm trying to escape into my comfort zone. Murder, I'm comfortable with. BDSM, I'm not. I force myself to keep my green-metal-picnic-table knowledge to myself as our waitress arrives, bringing another round of beers.

As she sets down their drinks, I watch the disconcertingly quiet and pale young man. He has strawberry blond hair and wears a pink shirt and aviator glasses with yellow lenses. Like Al, he's attended BDSM campouts. Occasionally, he gives a grin of knowing as Al reminisces.

The pallid nerd sits in stark contrast to the BDSMer on his right—a dark-haired beefcake in a tight T-shirt. He's been in the Lifestyle for fifteen years, he offers, only upon my query.

Despite the two silent men, a silent Magick, and an ill-at-ease Suzy, the conversation with Al flows smoothly from BDSM to his favorite movies—*An Officer and a Gentleman* and *A Civil Action*—from fantasies of seeing Diane Sawyer in thigh-high black leather boots to home building and back to kink.

Al professes that when he was a contractor for Dell computers—in the days when Dell employed a mere 500 persons—250 of the company's employees were active in the world of BDSM.

"How do you know this?" I ask.

He recognized them, he says, because he'd seen them at kink events. Besides, since high-tech is a way of life for them, they don't hesitate to express their darkest desires over the net.

Gil, a data processing programmer, agrees. In his T-shirt and blue jeans, he appears to be the average nice guy . . . with enviably smooth skin. I move my hand to my face to try to hide my acne, as Gil tells me his favorite TV channels are Turner Classic Movies and A&E. He also says he's a submissive whose fetish is being kicked in the penis. Reflexively I jerk and reach toward my groin, as if I'm male and can feel his pain. But since Gil is the only person who seems willing to talk to me, other than Al, I keep my attention on him.

Gil was living in a California farming community when he drove to Los Angeles to try a session with a professional Dominatrix. He liked it, and he's been involved in BDSM ever since.

According to Al, residents in one out of seven homes practice BDSM in some form, whether they realize it or not. That gives one a whole new perspective when surveying the neighborhood, he jokes.

I have no idea if what he's telling me is anywhere near accurate. No one else I've asked has been able to give me an estimate of how many Americans are involved in BDSM, with the exception of Sadistic Bastard. He'd suggested that the number of Alt.com subscribers reflected a mere 20 percent of the actual U.S. practitioner base, which at the time would have put the total figure at just under 13 million.

· · · · ·

The more beer Al drinks, the more he focuses on me. The more he focuses on me, the more I feel Magick hating on me. Maybe it's my imagination. But then I find out that the chain wrapped around her neck—the one that I thought looked like costume jewelry—is her collar to Al, meaning she's his submissive.

Al's laughter breaks me out of my focused, fearful, magical daze as I hear him brag about his desire to see a local blonde television news anchor tied to a Saint Andrew's cross. "She's wild," he says. I'd heard rumors, but nothing like that. He then reels off the names of famous singers from the 1970s, the 1980s, the 1990s, and on into the 2000s who he claims are into BDSM.

"How do you know this?" I say.

"Their lyrics," he answers.

The beefcake nods in agreement.

Al orders another beer. As he does, this vanilla Diet Coke reporter suddenly realizes she's had more BDSM beer than she can handle for her very first time. It's like I've been knocking back BDSM shots so hard and fast that I hadn't realized the toll they were taking on me. Naked women bound and whipped. Nice-looking men wanting to be kicked in the penis. A local news anchor bound to a Saint

Andrew's cross. Seemingly every popular singer from the past three and a half decades into BDSM. A collared woman glaring at me. Al drinking more and more and sitting closer and closer. And that's when it hits. I can't take another sip of BDSM. I find myself climbing out of that metal mesh insane asylum picnic table. "I'm sorry. I've got to go. I have a conference early tomorrow." And I get the heck out of there.

Being alone in my car feels so good. Strapped into its black leather driver's seat, I can breathe again. Safely . . . slowly . . . breathe.

Chapter 15

· · · · ·

"i'll have you know in my quest to get laid, i posted on craigslist, women seeking men last night and have since received over 100 responses," Jessica wrote. "sorting through this shit is ridiculous. so let me take a moment from that madness of married men, 55 year olds, and enormous penis shots to respond to you."

I'd emailed Jessica a list of more than fifty questions, but with that intro, I didn't care about the answers to my fifty questions. I wanted to know about her Craigslist men. But she told me nothing about them. Instead, she expounded on the differences between orgasms and orgasmic paralysis, which I'd asked her to explain.

"orgasms are a quick sort of bolt. the buildup is there but the release is quicker. paralysis is a buildup that sometimes can impede an orgasm. it's like i get so worked up i can't just find that release, it gets stuck behind the paralysis. but the paralysis can be overwhelming, like, please, stop touching me now, i can't take it any longer, get your tongue away from my clit. it can be too much. i can't give myself paralysis. i wish i could. but ultimately, i prefer the orgasm."

Part of me pondered her words—her descriptions. Another part of me, well, I just couldn't think about such. About orgasmic paralysis. About orgasms. The subject was too elusive.

But it stayed in my brain for the next three days. That's when Jessica returned for round two of answering my questions and mentioned that she'd had a face-to-face meeting with one of her Craigslist responders. That meeting—just the day before—had turned into a body-to-body encounter.

". . . had a lot of sex. it was fun. i am not looking for anything serious, just some good loving. and now i'm sore. i am very trusting of people and one day this may get me in a lot of trouble but so far, so good."

To my great frustration, Jessica still didn't tell me about her Craigslist sex; she told me what "kinky shit" she thought about during sex.

"oh, geez. this is perhaps where i get most embarrassed when discussing sex. ummm, i like to think about bestiality (how do you spell that?) and incest. not on myself, but just setting a scene with strangers and having it happen. but everyone gets off and everyone enjoys themselves. i have figured out that in order for me to have an orgasm with someone else i have to set a scene in my mind—some dad fucking his daughter or something illicit like that and right when they're about to get off in my brain is when i get off. this bothered me for a while, this technique, but who cares? i win, the person i'm with has gotten me off and they think they're a champ so i'll take it."

I ignored Jessica's mentions of bestiality and incest because I didn't want to think about her thinking about such. The "kinkiest" sex I wanted to think about was Craigslist. But the only additional mention she made of that was when she answered my question about the wildest sex she'd ever had: "well. yesterday was insane. the older i get, the better it gets."

Was she sending me into the journalist's form of orgasmic paralysis? Stuck in the anticipation of the unanswered question?

She talked about other encounters she considered wild, including performing fellatio on a former boss—at his desk, with the office door open, and a second time in a storeroom on top of the sacks of flour.

She discussed her self-described fence-sitting over her sexual orientation. "it feels like bullshit. like, why can't i make up my mind? . . . it would just be easier to choose one or the other. so many of my friends have thoughts on where i'll end up, who i'll end up with. i have no idea. right now i appreciate the easiness of guys—women can be so complex. . . . women require more conversation, more investment. i think about the lack of sex my ex girlfriend and i had and i have never, ever had that happen with a dude. and i don't want that shit to happen ever again." She particularly pointed out that straight girls were high-maintenance. "but," she insisted, "i refuse to rule anything out, anyone out."

She told me about her parents. "my mom was affectionate with me, but not over the top. my dad, no, never." She added, "i always used to thrive on not being touched—used to think it was cool to be so hard-core. fuck that. i love touching people, loving being touched—i think it's essential."

I paused on that line. My thoughts tumbled with confusion. Part of me so wanted touch, and part of me so didn't. And neither had a thing to do with orgasms. It was just simple touch—like fingertips on the arm.

I turned back to the computer screen.

"suzy, good god. this has been fun. anything else, please let me know. if not, send me the dirt on this here book and keep me updated as to anything pertaining to it."

Sadness washed over me. I felt Jessica was saying good-bye, and I didn't want her to leave. We'd been in constant contact for three weeks, and in so many ways, she was those fingertips on my arm.

When I'd gotten emotionally overwhelmed by the number of penis photos I was receiving, I'd turned to Jessica, because I didn't feel I could turn to my shrink. Jessica didn't shame and berate me over them, like my shrink had. She'd made me laugh.

"jesus, such a male ego thing. i find penises more comical than hot. i mean, they have their own agenda, they can stand up, whee, it's like a toy. i always just want to flick them with my fingers."

In my mind, if not my heart, Jessica was a friend I needed to help me through this journey. I clicked on an attachment she'd included. It was a photograph of her with her mother. They stood shoulder-to-shoulder, perhaps even touching. Thick strands of rich gray hair blew into her mother's eyeglasses.

Jessica's dark hair was tied against the back of her head so that it appeared short. Her nose was cute but prominent like a parakeet beak. A messenger bag was slung across her chest slicing her banded-neck-and-sleeve T-shirt at a forty-five-degree angle. A sweet little smile revealed straight, white teeth. Like her mother, she looked like a nice person—a cute, quirky, college student who would blend in on any Middle America campus.

Less than twenty-four hours later, I broke down and emailed her. "Okay, okay, I'm a typical needy female. Can we communicate more? If so, dang it, girl, tell me all the details about the guy you met from Craigslist. I mean details."

"we can communicate til the end of time," she answered.

And there I had my simple touch of fingertips on the arm.

· · · · ·

Three days after posting on Craigslist, Jessica walked into an Atlanta bar. She was so nervous that she'd changed her clothes ten times before finally pulling on a pair of tight jeans and a black tank top. A bit of feminine lace edged the tank's V-neckline. The bottom of the tank crept up her waist, just above the band of her jeans, revealing a glimpse of the tattoo on her stomach. She let her hair hang long, full, and curly across her shoulders with the intention of turning heads. Her eyes fluttered with a touch of shadow, which she rarely wore.

She eased over to a man in a long-sleeved, white shirt that accentuated his tan. He wore blue jeans that led down to a pair of flip-flops. She hated flip-flops. "Before I say anything dumb, are you Ralph?"

He was.

Jessica sat down, stealing repeated glances at his hands, trying to correlate his hand size to his organ size. Ralph was one of the few men who had not sent her a penis photo, which was one of the reasons she'd chosen him. Another was that he could spell.

They talked about life, his work, that he was nine years older than she. Jessica had no problem with that. She liked older men.

They did a shot of tequila. She grew tipsy. She wanted to. It made her feel more at ease—sexually at ease, that is. As they left the bar, Ralph rubbed her back. That was another reason she'd chosen him—he'd talked about giving good back rubs. She also liked that he was taking control.

They drove to his apartment. They walked his dog. As they walked, Ralph kissed Jessica. She thought that was sweet. Returning to the apartment, they started "going at it" on his couch. They moved to the bedroom where he massaged her back, before he performed oral sex on her anus, followed by traditional oral sex and intercourse. "Can I get involved?" she asked.

"Absolutely," he said.

Still, she didn't orgasm. She hadn't yet reached her needed comfort level.

They had anal sex, and she was glad she'd been practicing with a dildo since she'd never had "serious anal sex with a dude."

They took a cigarette break and stroked each other. She liked that, too—that he didn't "get all weird about touching or any sort of intimacy post sex." They shared dinner, and Jessica was ready to leave.

Ralph invited her to watch a movie. Before he started the flick, they walked the dog again. Once more, he kissed Jessica in the courtyard. She slipped down his jeans, "and gave him a blowjob. alright. fortunately, no one walked by." At least she didn't think so.

They "sort of" watched the movie and then had sex on his

couch. She got involved again; this time, she came. They cuddled.
He said, "You can spend the night."

In her mind, Jessica said, Why?

. . . . .

Ralph emailed her an "it rocked" thank-you. "so i emailed him back
and we're going to hang out tuesday."

In the meantime, there were others Jessica wanted to meet. One
described himself as a "wealthy sugardaddie"—six foot three, 205
pounds, and worked out every day. He thought Jessica sounded
perfect. "why not? his emails indicate some intelligence and (i can't
help it) i'm intrigued by a sugar daddy," she said.

"so who knows? i have to find out. this whole process is a game
to no end. i am being careful, being safe, not meeting anyone in a
non-public arena first, not giving out work info or address or anything like that."

She closed with "please ask me questions. i feel, despite having
never met you, that you are my confidant in this situation with all
this shit. my friends have a tendency to think i'm a bit out of control
but i swear, if you ever met me, i am as down to earth as they come.
i just like having a covert sex life."

Apparently this bond I felt with Jessica went both ways, but
what Jessica didn't know was that I was worried about her. Though
random sex with Internet men made me nervous—and she'd just
removed her Craigslist posting "because enough already"—I was
less concerned about that than her safe sex practices. In my fifty
questions to her, I'd specifically asked if she worried about STDs.

"i worry about them constantly," she'd replied. "yet it doesn't
stop me from carrying on."

She never mentioned condom use with Ralph, so I specifically
asked her about it.

"we used condoms for regular sex, not anal sex."

Figuratively, I shivered. While Jessica was going to bed with

Ralph, I was going to bed with approximately 185 pages of Centers for Disease Control statistics on STDs. According to the CDC, more than half of all Americans will eventually get an STD. Getting any sort of an STD increases one's chances of contracting HIV/AIDS. Yet only 14 percent of men and 8 percent of women think they're at STD risk.

"i'm wondering if i should be more concerned about this," Jessica wrote.

Yes! The number of documented STD cases in the U.S. was increasing significantly. And a new syphilis epidemic was spreading across the nation. If left untreated, syphilis, like HIV, can kill.

But Jessica had decided not to worry about STDs. "otherwise I would never sleep at night."

And I kept my *yes!* and STD information to myself—that breach-of-professional-ethic thing again, letting her know I cared.

· · · · ·

Over three days, Jessica met with four Craigslist men.

She rejected the first because she could smell his breath over the table. She rejected the second—the sugar daddy—because she realized she was too smart to have one. She rejected the third because she wasn't attracted to him, though she accepted his offer to go to his house and smoke pot.

They got to his house, smoked some weed, and he went to the bathroom to brush his teeth, presumably in preparation for sex.

And I thought about how people shouldn't brush their teeth or floss their gums before sex; they should gargle, because the toothbrush and the floss nick the gums leaving tiny open wounds that can be invaded by HIV. Random thoughts like that fill one's brain when one goes to bed with CDC STD stats.

He walked out of the bathroom, and Jessica stated, "I can't do this."

To use her word, she booked it out of there.

She went over to Ralph's. They had sex—oral and anal. They watched some lesbian porn, and they had more sex. Jessica enjoyed it, but she wanted more. She wanted an emotional connection.

"though i said specifically in my posting that i'm not looking for that, it is true that it helps. i like having sex, i like having sex with ralph because it's fun and i get off, but it's not blowing my mind."

Jessica was supposed to meet a few more men, but . . .

"i think the whole cl posting was valid and i don't regret doing it but it's definitely made me realize what i'm going after. it's also made me realize that i can't be as casual about shit as i'd like to think i can be."

She'd already told me that she didn't think she could "fuck some different dude every night. i can be casual but that's too much."

"i've also noticed that half of what i like so much is the tension, the possibility that maybe yes, this could happen, or maybe not. when it's a given, that's half the battle over. i live for the build-up."

"ralph's coming over on tuesday. we're going to handcuff each other to the porch i have here and go at it. still still still suzy, i wonder what exactly these guys find attractive in me. is it because i appear to be easy? am i just a cum depository? my boobs?"

Like Jessica, I always want to ask what anyone sees in me. And though that question forever lingers on the tip of my tongue, I think, I hope, I keep it to myself. I fear I'll appear too desperate and insecure if the words are actually released, that they'll then know that that's the real me, and they'll turn away. As an old TV ad used to say, "Never let them see you sweat."

"i would like to reach a point with him, which i hope happens, when i just feel more relaxed around him," Jessica said. "so now i'm just trying to decide what, if anything else, i want to do with these remaining guys. i will absolutely keep you updated."

• • • • •

Jessica did see Ralph again. He didn't handcuff her as promised, which irritated her. They didn't have anything to talk about, and the resulting, extended silences annoyed her. Worst of all, he never spoke her name, which made her feel like a whore.

"so I think I'm done with that."

Besides, there was Ryan, a thirty-five-year-old, recently divorced English teacher who'd sent her "some fairly ballsy naked pictures." But Jessica would have to tell me about him later, she said. She had to go to work. "hope you're well."

I wasn't.

Chapter 16

· · · · ·

"I am so battling depression and am so losing," I wrote Lola, my psychiatrist friend. "I phoned my shrink today and asked if I could up my Lexapro."

It wasn't Jessica who got to me. Not at all. It wasn't the one-on-one with my sex freaks that got to me, either. It was the *en masse*. Six months of *en masse*. There were so many of these people that I'd lost count of how many. A hundred maybe? At least. I had a foot-high stack of printed-out emails, and that didn't include everyone with whom I'd communicated.

In particular, it was the *en masse* men who got to me. There were so many of them that I was getting them mixed up. I'd think I was emailing Richard when I was emailing Dick. I'd phone Randy and ask him questions that were meant for Hung Like a Horse . . . or Moose . . . or whatever. Maybe that's why I was getting them mixed up. They all had the same names, usually having something to do with their ginormous endowment. Come on, guys—show some originality! I apologized to one man for not recalling what he'd said, and he told me that's because he and I had never spoken!

Then there were the number of cheating married men who claimed they were good guys and it was all their wives' faults. And the number of married men who yearned to be with and sought men. How was that their wives' faults? Maybe it was trying not to be judgmental that was getting me so down. Add to that the nonstop bombardment of penis photos. And the loneliness. Oh, my gosh, the loneliness.

Why, oh, why did Jessica always seem to lighten my mood?

She liked Ryan. He called her by name. He asked her questions. He treated her like a person, not just a sex object. He opened a bottle of wine. He asked, "Do you want me to kiss you?"

They kissed and kissed some more before they eased into the bedroom and had oral sex and intercourse. Still, Jessica didn't climax; she had a bout of orgasmic paralysis. Her body was too exhausted from too many days of sex and masturbation—at least that's what she told herself. But Jessica was also worried about how she couldn't relax, and she was really really really trying to relax. Her brain started reeling and she couldn't stop it. It was like she was thinking so hard about having an orgasm that that very hard thinking prevented her from coming. There just had to be a way of letting it go.

"How many times did you come?" Ryan asked.

Jessica lied.

"it seems so ridiculous that i spent the entire weekend having sex," she wrote me. "i'm trying to figure out if i need to slow my roll, if i should be feeling like a slut (what is that? such stigmas attached to women having sex and liking it) for two dudes in two days but i really feel until the end of time that [since] no one else is going to do this for me, i have to take matters into my own hands."

· · · · ·

The word "judgmental" again filled my brain.

I once had a friend who had two guys in one day. We had a fight about it. I told her I was worried about her getting STDs. I was really worried that she was a slut. I didn't want that for her, and I didn't want a slut for a friend.

But with Jessica, with my sex freaks, I had mixed emotions. Part of me wanted them to be safe and healthy. To me, healthy didn't include random sex with strangers one met over the Internet. Hell, it didn't even mean random sex with strangers one met anywhere. Then again, I enjoyed peeking into their lives. What am I saying? I enjoyed ripping back the velvet drapes and standing there like a ghost living through them. They had the guts to do the very things I never could.

I soon realized, though, it wasn't just a matter of guts. It was a matter of desire.

Jessica planned on having her very last Craigslist date the following night. "i just want to find a guy worth keeping in touch with," she said.

I thought about that. In fact, I thought about everything she'd written me. Everything so many had written me. All the talk of orgasms and lovers. Having many of one and unable to have even one of the other. Especially when it came to lovers—the inability in both men and women to find that one person, that one partner, who totally "gets" you. No matter what anyone said, they *all* seemed to want that.

But I still didn't. That's what I mean by it wasn't a matter of guts. It was a matter of desire. What was wrong with me that I could *not* desire having that one person in my life—that one person who I connect with mentally, spiritually, physically, and emotionally? I absolutely did *not* want that connection. I could not even fathom lying in bed with someone, hugging them, holding them, and connecting with them throughout an entire night and into the next morning. Letting them see the living, breathing, me. Heart and soul. Letting me need them. I could not go there. It did not seem to be in my being.

And maybe that's why I so cared for my sex freaks. I knew I'd never find that in them. They weren't safe in their sex practices. And that very lack of safeness made them safe for me—the wraith-like Victorian voyeur.

Chapter 17

• • • • •

"I like sweet sex."

A friend of my mother's said that to me well over a decade ago. In fact, she told me that more than once as we sat around the big, round coffee table in my mother's women's wear store. My mom's friends used to gather around that table, drink coffee, and gossip each Friday afternoon while my mother hemmed their garments or showed them the perfect shoes to go with that perfect dress. I'd sit there with a bottle of Coke, a Keebler pecan Sandy on a paper napkin, and flip through *Vogue*, while slowly scooching back my chair to avoid her friends' cigarette smoke. But I didn't want to scoot back so far that I couldn't hear. I loved being around these women.

That "sweet sex" day, they were talking about books. My mother's friend, one of three women I thought of as a second mom—and the only adult in my life who encouraged me to date—looked at me and said she loved Danielle Steel novels. I jokingly shivered and gagged. Danielle was too gooey for me. That's when my mother's friend said she loved sweet sex, which led her to talking about French kissing. At that, my mother seriously shivered, gagged, and pronounced French kissing gross. I didn't say anything. But I thought about that when I started communicating with Rex.

· · · · ·

At six feet, four inches tall and with salt-and-pepper hair, Rex could have been a character in a Danielle Steel novel. He described himself, though, as an overweight, middle-aged, married man who was a daily visitor to AFF, which is where we met.

"Frustration and boredom with my sex life at home" sent him to AFF, he said. "My wife is prudish and I like more than just the same thing again and again. I love her very much."

His lines were all ones I'd heard more times than I could count.

Then he said, "And we have talked about our sex life."

Now, that line stopped me. It was something I rarely heard.

"But it's just not that important to her."

Again, we were back to clichés. Rex, however, offered me specifics: "She doesn't like to French kiss. There is no oral either way. . . . Cum to her is 'gross,' and after I orgasm, she runs to the bathroom to clean herself up. For her, once a month is plenty. This doesn't even come close to doing it for me."

Rex had been a member of AFF in the website's infancy—when AFF had a mere one hundred thousand subscribers and he was single. Back then, he enticed and lured the women by chatting with them, making sure he got to know them on a personal level, and learning what they liked sexually. He hooked them by writing sex fantasy stories based on their individual desires and strategically never rushing them into meeting him in person.

I thought about my friend's desire for sweet sex.

"If I played it right," Rex wrote, "I could get them very excited about meeting me finally and almost always had sex on the first meeting."

Though what Rex wrote me could be interpreted as braggadocious come-ons, I took them as matter-of-fact answers to my questions. Then again, maybe they revealed his adeptness at never rushing a woman.

His past success at AFF motivated his return to the site when he became a sexually frustrated married man.

Rex's AFF profile emphasized that he was "a very good listener," had "a very good imagination," and that he loved to role-play. It also stressed that he was looking for friendship, not just a "fuck buddy." As proof, Rex told me he had five women on his Yahoo! Messenger list that he'd known at length, some almost ten years. "I usually have to sign on as invisible on Messenger because if they see me on they will message me right away if they are alone and want me to call them."

Typically they were older women because he refused to deal online with women who claim to be under thirty. "Women below that age, when they want phone [sex], invariably will play until they cum and then hang up on me before I get off. I'm sexually frustrated enough without having to add that to the mix."

And typically the women were married.

"I'd say I've always been pretty sleazy. I slept with A LOT of married women when I was younger, having a few relationships along the way, living with a couple of women. Mostly being interested in anything that was interested in me up until the mid to late '80s when people realized that AIDS was starting to run rampant. I started being more careful after that, but still had numerous affairs with married women."

I eventually learned that Rex had had a backseat affair with a much older woman from my hometown, one who'd occasionally shopped at my mother's store. I say backseat because they always had sex in the backseat of the woman's car. By then, Rex had experimented with role-playing and light bondage—handcuffs—as well as blindfolds and paddles.

So much for sweet sex.

When Rex realized he could combine role-playing with phone

sex, he was the one who was hooked. To him, phone sex was "much hotter" than watching a woman masturbate on her Web camera.

I pointed out to him that reputedly men are more visual than women; therefore it seemed that watching a woman on a Web cam would be more enticing to him than talking.

"It's like acting," he said. "You can be just about anyone you want. . . . And as far as visual, I can close my eyes during phone role-play and I am there."

There? I couldn't even be *there* during real sex. I had a tendency to float out of my body, hover at the ceiling, and watch. And no, I didn't mean that as another ghost reference. It's just what happened.

· · · · ·

Rex loved to create the scenario of the "neglected wife next door" and imagine what he called "serendipitous sex"—meeting someone in public and having sex with them "RIGHT THEN." Though in real life he preferred one-on-one sex, in phone sex he liked to weave in "a gangbang scenario for a woman who fantasizes about that." Women who were, in his words, "insatiable sluts" were a "huge turn on" for Rex. "I love to hear about how many guys they have phone fucked that day, or cybered with, or whatever. . . . And it's even hotter when I can get her to cum and cum and cum until she actually has had enough."

Rex utilized not only AFF but Yahoo! chat to meet those "sexually frustrated married" women, though in their profiles they didn't necessarily admit they were married. According to Rex, they "are just looking for some affirmation that they are still sexy women." In other words, he was finding the same women as J.D.

Only Rex's women were located all over the nation. And he *only* had phone sex with them—in the daytime, while their spouses were at work. He used prepaid phone cards to make the long distance calls so that his working wife would never find a telephone bill to wave in his face as proof of infidelity. Rex had inherited enough money to live comfortably, so he worked as a self-proclaimed

Mr. Mom, doing the grocery shopping, cooking, laundry, and housecleaning, and driving the stepchildren to school.

Rex and I were in our fourth day in a row of "talking" when he noted: "It is astounding to me how many women want to role-play the daddy/daughter fantasy. While I love this fantasy, it never involves little kids. And while there are some women out there that I've talked to who want to role-play a seven-year-old, this just creeps me out beyond belief. The fantasy usually is the girl home from college after her first year/semester, or the high school senior coming home drunk for the first time, getting a spanking and going from there."

I thought about Jessica. I didn't want to. I thought about Siouxsie Ramone.

Rex said he wasn't stretching the truth when he admitted he's had phone sex a few thousand times, sometimes three times a day. "I've had women leave an open phone line next to the bed and let me listen in while hubby fucks them, and him not knowing that I am. I have a friend now who wants to listen in while I have phone sex with another woman. She can't get enough of this. I'm hoping to get some as I sit here and write to you."

And he offered to me, "If you want to talk on the phone at some point, that would be fine, too. If not, just let me know what else I can do. Believe it or not, I'm not really one to talk about myself, so this has been interesting."

That was another line I'd heard more often than I could count—"I'm not really one to talk about myself." But as Rex, the self-professed "very good listener" knew, people readily confess their deepest secrets when talking to someone who truly wants to hear what they have to say . . . *and* who listens without judgment.

I thought about my shrink.

Cock shots—that's what I now called penis photos, despite the fact that the word "cock" had never before been part of my vocabulary. And I liked that I could use the word without jumping out of my body.

But that easiness wouldn't last long.

Chapter 18

· · · · ·

The day is hot, muggy, miserable. And I'm edgy, to put it mildly.
I'm meeting Albert again. Alone. And the Draught House, which
he picked, is too kinkily perfect. It feels like an eighteenth-century
dungeon—nineteenth-century at best. The lighting is darker than
the ale that's served. The air stinks of smoke and is uncomfortably
frigid, especially considering the heat outdoors. I peer through the
gloom, trying to find a seat with a bit of illumination. I need light
for my note-taking and my psyche. Perhaps more for the latter than
the former.

I see a table next to a tiny, dust-shrouded window. I literally plop
down; the seating's so low that the tabletop bumps up to my breasts.
I feel I'm being prepped for torture. I sit in uncomfortable silence.
There is no music—only the hum of refrigeration.

The silence breaks when two women ask for the nonsmoking section. There isn't one. A man reading a graphic novel lights up a smoke.
I'm not sure it's tobacco. Finally, the music's flipped on and Al arrives.
It's been two weeks since the munch, but this happy hour is starting
out the same. He orders a beer while I sit with my Diet Coke. This
time, though, I have my protection—my recorder. I click it on.

As a teenager, Al says, he built a lawn mowing business. That was about the same time he discovered that he liked to pinch his girlfriends' nipples. The girls wondered why. He didn't know why.

In his twenties, he sold his business, gambled away half its profits in Atlantic City, and moved to Dallas where he got into the restaurant business, to use his words. In fact, he became a waiter. Working at the same restaurant was a tall, blond, blue-eyed, fit, and assertive waitress, five years his senior. After hours, they went to her house and played chess. After a month of doing that, she turned to Al and informed him she didn't have him in her house until five-thirty in the morning just to play chess. They started sleeping together.

The third time they had sex, he asked her about her ex-boyfriend.

"Mason's just too vanilla," she answered. "All he wants to do is get laid. I want to push. I want to explore. Mason would never take me down to the pool and fuck me in the pool on a Saturday afternoon with thirty other people around. I have the idea that you would."

Are you nuts? Al thought.

Two Saturdays later, as she sat on Al's lap in the pool, he eased her bikini bottom aside to have sex in front of forty people, he says.

They moved in together; she taught him about sex toys, spanking, role-playing, dress-up, and bondage—of his testicles. Some nights he'd come home to find her dressed in boots and a leather cape and holding a whip.

"Get back outside, take your clothes off, crawl in here," she'd order.

The next night, he'd come home to find her blindfolded and chained to the bed.

"There were no defined roles," he says.

The relationship was short-lived. Al relocated to Austin and married a vanilla wife, who told him he was free to explore on his own. He did. They divorced.

As Al speaks, I nod and "uh-huh" every word he says. But while I'm nodding and "uh-huh"-ing, I'm questioning the veracity of his tale. For one thing, how did this woman chain herself to the bed? Maybe only her legs and one arm were chained. But my mind pictures her bound spread-eagled, unable to move. If she could have moved, what was the point?

I don't reveal my doubts to Al. I know if I do, he'll stop talking, and I want him to keep talking. He's my best in-person BDSM source. So I look into his face as though I'm enraptured.

With his hand wrapped around his second beer, he notes that "we in the Lifestyle" revel in the words "pervert," "perversion," and "kinky." "We are perverts," he pronounces. "Now, do I feel I am? Do I feel I'm perverted in a negative connotation? No, I don't. I feel pretty honored that I can be considered this."

I ask if he resents people from the vanilla world calling him a pervert.

"My ex-wife called me a pervert, okay. I laughed that off. I think *me* calling her vanilla is a worse insult than her calling me a pervert."

As the alcohol seeps into his brain, Al begins to lecture— submissiveness is not accepted in our society, only dominance is, men will tell many people about their submissive fantasies, but they won't fulfill them, that's the difference between Dominants and submissives. "Dominants will act."

I mention that many of the men I've spoken to want to be submissive with another straight male.

Al professes that society teaches that it's normal for women to have bisexual tendencies, but not for men. Yet both men and women start from an egg and sperm and have just one chromosome of difference. "And now you're telling me that because I have a penis and you have a vagina that we can't have bi fantasies? That's absurd. That's absolutely absurd."

"So have you ever had the fantasies or the action?" I say.

"I have had the action. When I was submissive to a Domme, that was part of her deal . . . bi male butt."

At that, Al gets up to go get another beer. I stare at the old men talking and the young men smoking, working on their computers, and playing darts as I think about where I want to go in my conversation with Al. But it's Dominant Al who directs the conversation when he returns with his third beer.

"I think the divorce rate in America has a lot to do with sexual compatibility," he says.

I'd certainly heard from enough people to believe that.

"The biggest thing is that they don't know how to convey it to the spouse. Maybe if they knew how to convey it—to talk to the spouse—they could get it done."

I don't even realize that I'm agreeing with what Al's saying because all I can think on is that Al's a nice guy through beers one and two, but with beer three, he commences to pontificate greatly.

"If the guy wants to wear women's panties, what's a little kink? If you married the guy and you're with him for seven years . . ."

I'm beginning to feel he's droning.

"We're so busy with everything in our lives that we don't pay attention to our primal sexual alliance. . . . If there's one thing in the D/s Lifestyle that sticks out more than anything else, it's communication. I think we do it better."

Pontificating? Hell. Blowhard is the word. So I ignore a lot of what he's saying, but I hear him proclaim that the D/s communicate better because they have so many avenues of communication—such as a Master ordering his slave into the closet because she doesn't have His desired dinner.

Oh, geez.

Yet, he says, the divorce rate is higher in the BDSM community than in society at large.

"Why is that, if you're communicating so?"

"Well, because you have different facets of relationships." Two people can be friends, lovers, spouses, and parents. "Now you add Dom/sub, there's another facet. Is that going to make that relationship more successful or is it going to give it one more facet for it to fail? That's what it does—it gives it one more facet to fail."

It seems to me that he's contradicting himself—people divorce because of lack of communication, BDSMers communicate better, but their divorce rate is higher than the norm.

"I think what I do as a Dominant, I read my submissive," he says. "I read her physical actions as well as her mental actions as well as her emotional reactions to things."

Obviously, he isn't reading me.

I want to stop the droning and pontificating, so I try to change the subject. I ask him about a recent kink event he attended.

"Magick sucked my cock for a little bit while I was flogging her. Just a little bit because I wanted to give her that because that's something she craves and wants to do that in front of other people."

The more Al drinks, the more I feel his words are a hand on my thigh, which he's waiting to see if I knock away or not. I'm determined to pass his test. Still, I contemplate how to make sure he knows this is just my job and not my desire, but before I figure that out, he stops to go to the restroom again and get a fourth beer. When he sits back down with me, he orates even more. If I were a cartoon character, my eyeballs would be spinning orbs—black-and-white spinning pinwheel orbs.

I ask him about slut training, something another one of my sources had mentioned and I hadn't really understood.

"In graphic elaboration, they're going to fuck who they're told, suck who they're told. They're going to do exactly what they're told to do to whoever they're told to do."

He proclaims orgasm control is his favorite form of play. "That is control at its top. You can tell somebody to come and they *do*. Or when they're ready to, you tell them 'you can't,' and they don't. That's control. Okay. . . . And is an orgasm sexual? Of course it is."

He claims he phoned a woman, asked her where she was—she was driving down the interstate—and then said to her, "Come."

"And she came. How can that happen if it's sexual? How to get her to that point is sexual. But it is control. With control comes responsibility. . . . If they're driving down I-thirty-five and you say 'you come right now' and they do it and hit somebody in front of them, you need to be responsible for that action," he laughs.

Al says just this afternoon he received a call from a woman he'd met online. She was driving down Interstate-35, when he told her to pull her ass into a parking lot, push her seat back, take off her shorts and panties, and stuff her panties inside her pussy.

He looks at me and says, "And she said she did. Now, do I know she did? No, I don't know she did. But she was getting really hot and wet over it."

"Here's the deal," he said to the woman. "To you right now this is sex. . . . But to me it's just a matter of me controlling you, so I want you to play with your clit with this hand and I want you to pull those panties out of your pussy very, very slowly. And when those panties pop out of your pussy, you come. This is not an option."

Again, he looks into my face and says, "And she did. I guess. She said she did. Now, can I trust her? I don't even know her. I've never met her. But she said she did. She said, 'God, that was awesome.'

"And why is it awesome? Why do you think it is awesome? Because she was sitting in a grocery store parking lot, with her shorts around her ankles, she's a hot chick, and she's got panties in her pussy and she's doing something sooo crazy. But if she did it— if she did it—and hopefully she got something from it, but it is control. It is what it is.

"And I asked her a couple of times, 'Anybody around you? Are your doors locked? Do you feel safe?' And one time she said, 'No, there's a bunch of people walking around.'"

He's turning red as he's telling me this.

"I said, 'Stop what you're doing. Let's stop. Let's just stop right now.' And she said, 'Oh, no. No. I'll just wait for them to go on by.'"

Once again, I'm not sure I believe his story, but I look at his red face and I believe he's turned on by it. So I ask to close off our conversation because pains are shooting up my right wrist and it aches from writing for so long. And that is the truth.

Al offers to get me a beer, which I turn down, and then he asks if I drink at all.

I know there's no way in hell I'm going to drink around this man. I want to make sure I'm the one in control of me. But I don't say that.

He goes to the restroom and then gets another beer. We talk some more. I'm getting uncomfortable. Very uncomfortable. I feel like he's moving closer and closer to me, while I try to millimeter away. I feel as though his hand truly is on my thigh. I feel like he's fantasizing the things he's going to do to me.

But I stay because I'm me—the teenaged girl who can't eke out the words to tell the married workman "don't touch me," the young adult who desperately needs to soothe her angry friend after he tries to stick his penis inside her, the woman who doesn't want to let the Dominant intimidate her and win, the professional journalist who doesn't want to offend and lose her best in-person BDSM source.

Al then tells me that if a woman phoned him and asked him to help her "get off," he'd do it. "It's the same as helping someone get gasoline." He says he'd want and expect the same from a female friend, and he tells me I'm sending out sexual vibes.

And that one line—that I'm sending out sexual vibes—is enough to make me stand to go. Because I know it's a lie. I am *not* sending out sexual vibes. Al stands, too, and he gives me a hug. It feels binding, not platonic. I don't like it. It's the most uncomfortable I've felt during all my research. But I don't tell him that. Again, I don't want to let him win, nor do I want to lose him as a source.

Instead, I drive home, power up the computer, and email Rose, telling her about the hug and the alleged sexual vibes. But I was working, that was all. "I'm always much more comfortable/relaxed when I'm working rather than in a social situation." And I'd let Al take that comfort away from me.

Chapter 19

· · · · ·

Typically, Coyote has an hour on his computer before his wife of thirty-five years comes home from work. That means he has to be alert, quickly search Alt.com, type rapidly—though he is a two-finger typist—and be ready to shut down everything as soon as he hears her enter the house. He thinks his wife is an angel. But as he sat at the computer one afternoon, he couldn't stop staring at the picture of the blindfolded woman whose hands were cuffed to her ankles. Her husband had invited Coyote to have sex with her.

Coyote had never done BDSM, and he figured the only way to learn whether he was into it or not was to try it. Switching to Yahoo! Messenger, he and the husband set up the rendezvous. They'd meet in Lampasas, Texas, a small ranching and hunting community less than forty minutes from the couple's home near Fort Hood military base.

On the appointed day, Coyote pulled on clean blue jeans, his work boots, and a fresh, nice shirt. He didn't like any odor. If he walked in and a woman stank, he was right out the door. He climbed into his navy blue pickup truck and checked his secret

*compartment behind the seat. There he stowed his cell phone,
which he called his "untraceable" phone because it was a
pay-as-you-go TracFone. That way there were no bills or phone
numbers for his wife to find. And though she knew he had the cell
phone, she couldn't use it. Coyote kept it locked with a code that
he had memorized. After all, the phone stored the numbers to his
sex contacts.*

*Hidden next to his phone was a Visa credit card, which his wife
didn't know about. He used it to pay for his Alt membership, as
well as AFF, and his sex rendezvous motel rooms. The Visa bill
went to his office, not his home, and he made payment with a
money order, not a check. The secret compartment in his truck
protected his condoms, too, which he certainly didn't tell his wife
about. Lastly, it hid his stash of Viagra, which "kept him in the
game" when he was "expecting a good long session." Coyote got
the drug from the Veterans Administration. That way his wife never
knew how many pills he had and how many he used, though they
made his face flush red. He swallowed back the little blue pill.*

*An hour later, Coyote pulled into Lampasas and parked at an
intersection next to U.S. Highway 190, the road he knew the couple would be taking. Coyote liked to arrive early and watch for his
sex partners, wondering if he could pick them out and wanting to
check them out before they checked him out. He watched the highway and the motel across the way. He was sure they'd register there.*

*His cell phone rang—they were running late, but they'd be there.
"We're going to get a room and then we'll call you back," the wife
said.*

*Coyote waited . . . and waited . . . and waited. The couple never
called. But as he sat in his vehicle, he observed a couple drive into
the motel parking lot. The man looked to be in his fifties and the
woman in her thirties, just like the couple he was supposed to meet.
Still, no call came. What the crap? He started his truck and drove
across the street and into the motel parking lot. He parked next to
the couple's car. And he waited.*

*The man walked out of a room, over to his car, stared straight
at Coyote, got into his vehicle, and drove off. Five minutes later,
Coyote's secret cell phone rang.*

"Man, we got in the room and the damn phone wouldn't work.
I had to drive five miles back down the road to get the phone
working."

"I was sittin' right next to you when you left."

Upon the husband's return, he walked over to Coyote's pickup.
"When you get in there," he said in a slight Northern accent, "you
can do whatever you want to her. She's yours. Give me just a few
minutes to get her ready and I'll give you a signal and come on in."

*A few minutes later, the husband opened his motel room door
and motioned for Coyote. Coyote walked in to find the husband
sitting fully clothed in a chair in the corner. The wife lay stretched
out on a double bed in a red negligee, a black blindfold over her
eyes, her hands cuffed, her feet shackled. Clamps hung tightly to
her nipples and clitoris. An array of toys was neatly laid out on a
second double bed. Coyote tried to eye them nonchalantly—more
clamps, a dildo, a few small whips.*

"Sit down," the husband said. "Have a beer with me." He
gestured toward his wife. "She's not going anywhere."

"Doesn't look like it," *Coyote mumbled, his lips barely moving.
He sat down and popped open a beer. He seldom drank before
having sex. That was something he saved for the last few minutes
of his drive home. But he had a cold one while he and the husband
small-talked and the wife lay silent and motionless on the double bed.*

Five minutes later, the husband again waved toward his wife.
"Here's the toys. There she is. Help yourself. Have fun."

*Coyote shed his clothes. He bent over the woman and licked
her just above her clit. He pulled off the clamp so that he could
nibble directly on her.*

"There's some more stuff there if you want to use it," *the husband said, indicating the toys, floggers, and what not.*

"I'll be honest with you," Coyote smiled. *"I really don't know what that stuff is or how to use it."* Sometimes, he could be a bit shy, even in his boldness. He rolled on a condom and penetrated the woman. Still cuffed and shackled, clamped at the nipples, and blindfolded, she couldn't see Coyote. His beard was graying; his face was ruddy with rosacea. Decades of beer had rounded his belly. A tattoo was inked into his shoulder.

The husband snapped pictures. The wife moaned. The cuffs and shackles slowly came off. The woman rolled over on her stomach. Coyote forcefully pulled back her hair and entered her from the rear.

"Fuck me harder," she whispered.

He tugged her hair tighter. The husband clicked off more photographs.

"Fuck me harder." The clamps fell off her nipples. *"Fuck me harder."*

Coyote didn't even notice when her negligee came off.

"Slap my ass," she begged. Her excitement dripped down her legs.

Coyote pulled out, took off the condom, stood up, and moved close to her face. She pushed off her blindfold, crawled on her hands and knees, and sucked on his testicles. He handled his penis, while the husband continued snapping pictures. Coyote shot his cum on her breasts. The husband photographed it, and the wife licked Coyote clean.

Afterward, Coyote took a shower, shared a second beer, and chatted with the husband.

The wife lay naked on the bed smoking a cigarette, as Coyote walked out the door.

. . . . .

Coyote timidly looks down at his plastic cup of iced tea as he tells me this.

We sit in a Whataburger restaurant, a fast-food place that I frequent too often but have chosen just because of that. Its employees will watch out for me.

Our first face-to-face meeting is awkward, comfortable, and relaxed, if that makes any sense. Coyote seems ill at ease. I think my looks do that to him in that it's apparent that he's somewhat attracted to me, which makes him unsure of how to act around me. So I'm working hard to make him feel comfortable, which makes me feel a bit awkward. But at the same time, we've communicated so intensely for two months via email that I think we both feel like we're friends. Maybe the awkwardness is just both of us trying to nonchalantly look each other up and down as we assess each other. I try not to stare at the tiny red veins that criscross his tanned cheeks or the way his T-shirt curves over his beer gut.

"You're staying pretty busy with this stuff, huh?" he mumbles through thin lips. "Is it interestin'?"

"Pretty interestin'," I say as I fumble with my tape recorder, making sure that it's working.

"Pretty interestin'?" he repeats, his accent pure Texas.

"It goes from interesting to sad to sometimes scary to funny. Just a little bit of everything." But I don't want to give him time to focus on me, so I zoom into saying, "So tell me how's the Internet working for you?"

"Good," he answers. And with goading he continues. "It makes it easy. Oh, there's a lot of people that are on there just talkin', you know, but I have met quite a few from off of there. It's kinda—you learn somebody from the inside out. It's kinda like learning somebody in reverse. Say, if I met somebody, I may have these desires and stuff, but they might not know it until I know them for a long time. With this, you know what they want before you ever actually meet 'em as a person. It's like eliminatin' all the small talk or whatever you want to call it."

"What is it that the women are usually wanting?"

"Everything."

We both laugh.

"I mean, everybody's a different individual. The women, maybe they're not gettin' enough at home. Or maybe their husband has a problem or something. And there's a lot of couples on there, too, that, you know, they like a threesome."

I ask him to tell me about some of his threesomes.

"One thing that I have learned is that a lot of times the male will be bisexual, you know, so you're there with the guy and the woman, basically. He may want to do something to you. He may not. It just depends. Like I said, everybody's different."

"So do you consider yourself bisexual?"

"I haven't done a man, no. Don't intend to. But I'm not saying that it couldn't happen if the situation was right. Like I said, every situation, every couple, every person is different. They want different things. You know basically what they're after when you meet. But then after you're with them a time or two, you kind of get a little more at ease with each other."

Coyote chews on his ice.

"The first time I was with them," he says, referencing a married couple he's been with, "I didn't know he was bisexual, you know. She kept making little remarks about what he might like to do to me. And finally I just told 'em go ahead. And, you know, after that he's done me a couple of times while she watches or—"

"When you say he did you, a blowjob or anal sex?"

"Blowjob," he says.

"Blowjob," I repeat.

"'Cuse me." He stammers nervously. "I'm from the old school. I don't like to use some words around a lady."

"I'm getting used to a lot of the words," I say, trying to reassure him.

"I just gotta get a little more easier about saying it."

"I'm sorry. I'm just sorta attacking you on this."

"I'm a little nervous, but I'll get over it," he timidly mumbles. "You know, I haven't told anybody about a lot of this stuff. You know, people I work with for years don't have any idea."

"See, that's one thing that has surprised me," I whisper, "is how many bisexual men I've run across. You know, they say it's trendy for women to be bisexual. But I am just *shocked*—I mean, no one would look at you and think—ever."

Put Coyote in a roadside bar with an old jukebox full of George Strait tunes and no one would pick him out as man who'd *ever* done *anything* sexual with another man. He is a Texas good ole boy complete with gimme cap that's embroidered with an American flag and a pickup truck covered in American flag decals.

"I enjoy it. It's adult pleasure. It's recreational sex, I think is what they call it. It's not—you don't have to tell the lady how much you love her and all this stuff and buy her lunch and supper and everything. You just meet and do what you have to do. So you step away. And I use protection. You know, with things going around like they are now days, you're just kinda asking for it."

"I'm glad to hear that, because so many people that I talk to don't."

"No, I'm pretty—That's one of my rules." And once again Coyote tells me that his wife is a very good woman, whom he loves dearly. "I wouldn't want to hurt her in any way whatsoever. This is just something I've got. You know, it's kinda like some people have a gambling addiction or something like that. I don't hunt. Don't fish. Only thing I hunt is something to play around with." He chuckles under his breath. "I surf the net. That's where I do my huntin'.

"Sometimes, it's hard to get out of the house. I have to make some kind of excuses about—well, just like today. If somebody was to say—if somebody saw us here or something, well, I wouldn't mind telling them you're working on a book, but not about sex. It's going to have to be like you're working on a post-traumatic stress syndrome book or something like that. You know, I've been diagnosed with that." It's from his service in Vietnam thirty years ago. "I mean, it's something that as you go through life, raising your family and everything, you do things that you feel bad about and you wonder why you did it, and now we're starting to find out—"

He was diagnosed just a year ago.

"And you can't go back and raise your family again. They say put the past behind you, but you can't go back and redo a lot of things."

I wonder if PTSD is why he pursues sex so much.

"No, not really."

"Just a man, huh?" I joke.

"'Cause I was that way before I went to Vietnam. . . . I guess it's the hormones. I don't know."

I can tell he's getting more comfortable with me. His constant laughter is more sincere than nervous anxiety. And, as for me, I can breathe with Coyote, unlike with Albert.

Three years out of Vietnam, Coyote married the woman whom he again describes as "a true person" and "a good woman."

"She gen-u-winely cares about people. She's an outstanding mother. She's perfect in every way, except she just dudn't enjoy sex like I do. . . . This has been going on for years, so if I don't initiate it, she could go months and months and months without anything. And that's another thing . . . to me part of the enjoyment is knowing that they want me, not that I'm taking it from them. I cain't do that. I could never do that."

From that, our conversation meanders to BDSM. "I just don't know why anybody would want to get the crap beat out of them, you know."

Yeah. I nod internally.

"I guess they've got their own reasons."

Inside, I'm shaking my head, wondering what those reasons are.

As he mentions a woman who wants to give him a blowjob, he brings up the topic of photographs. "Some of them like pictures. Some of them don't care for pictures."

"You mean pictures of you?" I ask.

"Of, you know, your endowment."

"Oh, okay," I say, followed by a long silence. *Penis pics.* "Do you go into the bathroom and take them or what?"

"Oh, yeah." He details how he goes into the bathroom, gets himself "good and worked up" and takes a picture of himself "—or even ejaculate. A lot of them like to see that stuff. Turns them on. . . . Some like them really wet."

He explains that many couples like to have photographs of what they've done with others. "They'll send these pictures to each other over the Internet or put them on their profile or something like that. But they don't want their face on there for obvious reasons, you know."

Yeah, I know, I think to myself. But, in fact, I can't imagine. I can't imagine letting someone take my picture like that and put it on the Internet. What about one's career? What about one's kids? What if somebody you know sees it and exposes you? That's certainly happened. But all I say to Coyote is "How do you make sure they don't get your face?"

"Trust. Mainly," he says. "You could meet somebody that could really do you a bad number if you're not careful. But most of the people, believe it or not, what they're doing sounds horrible, but they're really decent, honest, and caring people. They just have this deal for sex."

Coyote's not simply a good ole boy. He's also a good person who spends his free hours doing good deeds for the community, which in turn lands him in the newspaper and on television, where he's applauded for his help and heartfelt kindnesses.

"Before the Internet there was not that many ways to get out there, you know, and search for people. You could put an ad in a magazine or something and wait two or three weeks for somebody to write you back and maybe eventually trade phone numbers, but this, I mean, you can look 'em up. On a search, you can even put in there what you're looking for, you know, age factors and hair color, anything, and have a search come up with just those people that meet those requirements."

I think six feet tall, not more than six feet, two inches; blond; blue or green eyes; perfect teeth; beautiful smile; firm but not bulky, lean but not skinny; Christian; liberal; workaholic; travels a lot, so that I don't have to deal with him all the time; hysterically funny; ambitious—

"Of course, I'm getting up there where I'm not all that picky anymore."

I laugh.

"You know what I mean?" He smiles. "The older you get the less responses you get, especially when you're married. A lot of them don't like to mess with married men, you know."

Married, so that I don't have to deal with him all the time. Married, so that I don't have to worry about him wanting to get married. "Why is that? Because I would guess that would be easier," I say.

"Well, sometimes there's a lot of scheduling conflicts. Married men cain't get out just ever' time a woman wants him, you know. Some of 'em put in their profile 'need to be available upon a phone call' or something like that. I mean, she may get hot pants and wants it right now. And a married man cain't just drop the phone and say, 'Baby, I'm going to the store. I'll be back in five hours.'"

Five hours! Holy shit! More like five minutes. . . .

"You know what I mean? So the Internet makes it a whole lot more convenient."

I watch him check out a girl as she walks past us. She's young, stunning, brunette, shapely. Did I say young? Very young, not illegal, but very young.

"I can't help it," he smiles.

"That's okay. It doesn't bother me." And it really doesn't. I like Coyote, but I'm not interested in him in *that* way.

Besides, when I looked at the girl, all I could think was *Sheesh, I wish I looked like that.*

"You know, my wife, when she's with me, I try to, you know, she gets a little aggravated at me sometimes. She's kind of a jealous type, too."

"Do you think she suspects at all?"

"No." He tightens his grip around his plastic cup. "I really don't." The ice in his tea jangles as he takes another gulp. He then sets the cup down on the Formica tabletop with a soft thud. "Sometimes she walks in when I'm on the Internet."

One time, she walked in and said, "How come every time I walk in here you're just looking something up or how come the screen is blank?"

He replied, "Well, because I'm always looking at crap. You know how this computer is."

With me, Coyote retreats to defense and emphasizes again that he's *tried* to get his wife to do *something* to make their sex life a little more exciting.

I let it go. After all, he's not my husband. "How often do you hook up with people?"

"It depends—mainly on when I can. Um, I have a better time getting loose during the day like this than on weekends 'cause my wife's working and I'm down here in Austin . . . so I know where she's at." Plus, when she's home on weekends, she wants to go with him wherever he goes. "Unless she goes and visits her mom and dad . . . then I can get on the phone and hook up with somebody pretty quick if I'm in the mood."

He's drinking his iced tea a lot faster now.

"Would you say you do it weekly? Or monthly?"

"I might do it twice a week." He sucks on an ice cube. "I might do it once a month." It all depends on when he's off work and when he has a Veterans Administration appointment. ". . . Because if I know I've got an appointment, which I usually know ahead of time, I'll try to set something up. . . . You've got to kinda take advantage of every spare minute you get, you know. Sounds bad, but . . ."

In truth, Coyote's sneaking around on his wife is somewhat of a new thing for him, three years due to the Internet. Prior to the Internet, he'd had one affair—with the wife of one of his "good friends"—plus numerous quick and free blowjobs from men. "You can go to any rest stop on the highway, especially late at night. You pull in there and go in there and go to the bathroom and about half the time there's going to be a guy in there wanting to play with you."

"Really," I say calmly.

"Yeah, and you know, they have their little signals, like they may scratch their self a little bit or something or look at you or they may glance down at cha and kinda make a little eye contact without saying anything and you can kinda look back and give 'em a nod or something like that and you go out to the car or the truck or whatever and let 'em have what they want. That's mainly what I did during the years of raising the kids. But I was very careful about that, too, because I damn sure didn't want to get caught and embarrass my family and everybody." He swirls and drinks his tea.

"So what would you do to take precautions?"

"Oh." He's quiet for a very long time, long enough for me to notice that the music in the background isn't country, for which I'm grateful. Finally, he says, "You just have to be careful and watch out. I mean, when you're sitting in a car in a roadside park somewhere, you kinda gotta be aware of who's walking around and doing what, you know. Of course, it's dark. Some of them have vans with dark windows and stuff like that. That's a good vehicle because you can get in the back of it and the people can't see in. And it doesn't matter if it's daytime or night. Or some of them have apartments. You can go to their apartment."

He gulps his tea again. It seems that every time we talk about blowjobs, he drinks more and more iced tea.

These days, he sets up his blowjob appointments through the Internet, where he's only an occasional paying customer at sites like AFF and Alt.com. People with free accounts—like me—can only answer emails. Paying customers can send emails and initiate contacts.

Coyote pays his $20 monthly fee and sends out maybe a hundred emails, expecting few responses due to his age and marital status. But once he makes several contacts and sets up a few meetings, he goes back to a standard, nonpaying membership.

"But, uh . . . after a few months or something, I'll be setting there looking at it . . . ," he shakes his ice in his cup, "and all of a sudden something will catch my eye, and I'll say, whoa, so I'll get my credit card out and activate my account and start answering some more ads." He shakes his ice again. "My wife went down to Houston a while back to see her folks, and I set there all day. Of course, my computer's not any speed demon. You sit and you wait and wait and finally, okay."

He keeps drinking that tea and I can hear that the cup's almost empty.

"Have you met anyone that you really like, that you'd want to be friends with?"

Coyote understands that I mean friends beyond sex.

"Oh, yeah, yeah. The main problem there would be explaining to my wife where I met these people, you know. . . . I was going to go spend the night with a couple in San Antonio one time, and I told her that one of my VA buddies was having a party. And I said his wife was going to be out of town, and I'm going to go over there and have a few beers, and if I have too many I'll just stay. . . . But, yeah, there's some of them—I mean they're good people. And a lot of them are pretty, uh, pretty well-respected in their communities and well-known people, you know, that, that, that the community has no idea what they're doing. And, I mean, it's a pretty high-class people I guess is what you'd call it."

I flip the page of my legal pad as I ask him to give me an example.

"People in politics," he says. A county tax assessor used to give him blowjobs. "And didn't help me on my taxes any," he grins and chuckles under his breath, "but we had a good time together."

They met at a party. The tax assessor's wife was there, too. As they were chatting, the assessor, who was older, mentioned that he couldn't drive at night, so he asked Coyote to drive him to Austin for meetings.

"He'd pay me like twenty bucks to drive him down here. And of course, one thing led to another and he got to messin' with me and he rented a room and just gave me a good'un."

As Coyote explains to me the one thing leading to another, his voice dries with apparent nervousness. "I was driving and he started talking about going to a party somewhere onetime where everybody got naked"—repeatedly, Coyote has to clear his throat—"and then he started talking about sex and being naked and everything to see what my reactions were. Of course, I knew—it didn't take me long to figure out what he was working towards."

Once a week for the next two or three months, their Austin sex trips continued.

Coyote clears his throat again before he tells me that the assessor gave him a blowjob in the tax office. "People would not believe everything that I've done. I don't—I cain't tell anybody for one thing." He lifts his plastic cup to his lips. "Sometimes, it's a wonder I ain't been shot."

A baby babbles in the background as Coyote tells me he could think about sex all the time "if I wanted to. In fact, I do—every time I see a woman. But, you know, I've always been that way. . . . Before I was even old enough to ejaculate, I was messing around on a swing set . . . trying to climb up the side of it, and . . ." He explains that when he was six or seven years old, he could get an erection by climbing a metal pole—his legs rubbing and holding the steel. "And *something* happened." He didn't know what it was. "But it damned sure felt good, you know." So he did it regularly. "I called it tickling myself. . . ."

*   *   *   *   *

As our conversation moves on, the thought of Coyote's "wonder" that he's never been shot returns as he tells me about meeting a police officer and his wife. As the cop undressed, he pulled out his pistol and laid it on the dresser. Coyote, frightened, stared at the gun and thought, *I hope this guy don't get mad easy—these people could pull some kind of crap on me, and how am I going to explain anything?*

"I think about things like that every once in a while . . . ," he says to me and laughs, barely revealing his teeth.

"Do you ever feel guilty about this?"

"Yeah, on occasion I do, but it passes. And the next time I get a little horny, well," he reaches for his tea, "I'll be right back on there again. Sometimes right after I get through leaving a place, I feel bad about it. I think I need to quit doing this, this is not right. And, like I said, give me a few days and I'm back on there searching.

"Not all the time I feel bad about it, but sometimes I do. I feel guilty and dirty and how could I do this to her, you know, things like that, 'cause it would really tear her to pieces if she knew what I was doing, and I wouldn't want that to happen for anything in the world. That's the reason I've gotta be so careful about who I'm with, when I'm with them, and you know, taking any unnecessary chances. Damn sure don't want no diseases."

"What about toys?" I say. "Where do you keep them?"

"I don't have any," he says. "The people usually furnish those if they want to use them. Maybe I should get some and let her find them," he laughs. "I don't know. Maybe that would help. You don't have any recommendations?"

I'm so discombobulated by his question that I can't form words. I only stammer.

He laughs.

"You're the first person who has gotten me to blushing," I say.

"Well, I'm just being me," he chuckles.

"Well, I like it. It's fine," I say, though I'm still stammering.

Then he says, "I'll be right back." But Coyote doesn't go anywhere physically, at least that I can see above the tabletop. He just turns so that his gaze can follow the pretty girl who's walking by us again.

"Okay, let me ask then, is there any particular type that you like?"

"I like dark-haired women."

Uh-oh. I feel myself panicking and grinning internally.

"Dark hair turns me on more than blond does. Nice breasts."

I feel him staring at my chest that has enlarged with my middle-aged weight gain.

"I don't mind a woman being a little bit plump—"

Oh, Lord, he is describing me.

"—but I don't like a real obese one, you know, although I have had some, which were pretty good, by the way. But I mean it's just kinda not my idea of a perfect woman. And I don't care about a perfect woman. All I want is a woman to have a good time and enjoy it with me, you know. I'm not perfect either, shit."

I wonder aloud if he'd be exclusive to his wife if she played the way he wanted her to. "Or would you still need other people?"

"I don't think I can be happy with just one woman," he says. "I need a variety. And I wouldn't say that just because my sex drive is that strong. I'm just saying that because variety keeps it more interesting."

That's why his computer is set up for two users. There's his wife's folder, and there's his. His folder is accessed via a password only he knows. And to retrieve his AFF mail, he has to click on a certain file, click on a certain message, click on a link, which finally takes him to AFF. Just in case he accidentally leaves on the computer where his wife could access it or he inadvertently leaves out his password, he deletes anything that's "questionable" and "everything that means very much."

"Hell, she may know everything about what I'm doing and I just don't know it, but I don't think so because she'd be stomping that little foot by the time I got home. Maybe more. Baseball bat or something."

When Coyote and I part that day, I leave him sitting in his pickup truck, his cell phone to his ear, a roadmap in his lap, finding his way to his next anonymous sexual encounter.

Chapter 20

• • • • •

Just before 8 P.M. on Friday the 13th, I jump in my car and race over to the east side of Austin to a neighborhood known for poverty, drugs, and violence. It's been a hectic day: 10 A.M. meeting with Coyote. 3 P.M. photo shoot for a magazine, during which the photographer told me about a dildo bar in San Francisco. The waitstaff, she said, served up dildos like cocktails on a tray. And now 8 P.M., SAADE—short for School for the Advanced American Dominant Education—and a seminar on the psychology of bondage.

Lord, what a life I'm leading.

I was invited to SAADE by Angela and Kai, a couple who contacted me more than two months before through Alt.com. Angela is bisexual, Kai is heterosexual, and Angela and Kai are kinksters *and* swingers. In their first email to me, they said, "We are both comfortable being observed & discussing our sexual experiences and feelings."

That phrase—"we are both comfortable being observed"—had made me uncomfortable. Would they want me to watch them have sex? Like J.D. did?

But J.D. had been a safe two hundred miles away and had disappeared from my email box before I could say yes. Angela and Kai were a not so safe thirty miles away.

And if Angela and Kai *did* want me to watch them have sex, what did they expect it to lead to? After all, I didn't know what they were into . . . except swinging . . . and kink . . . and she was into Wicca.

That completely freaked out this Christian.

All I knew about Wicca was what I'd seen in the media, after Wiccans had begun holding religious services at Fort Hood military base. Christians and congressmen had vehemently protested, proclaiming that Wiccans were devil-worshipping, animal-sacrificing witches who would destroy America and its military. The Christians and congressmen's arguments had been so vivid that I remembered them six years later. So when I'd read "Wiccan" in Angela's email, I thought "devil-worshipping, animal-sacrificing witches."

I asked Angela to educate me about her faith.

She'd tried most religions, she said. Her father had been reared Baptist, her mother Methodist. Both had become agnostics, but they'd allowed Angela to attend any church she wanted. None had felt right—none until she found Wicca.

"When I read for the first time about Wicca, it was like I had come home," she emailed me. "It spoke to me & I felt the presence of the Goddess—as I do right now as I write this." Wicca doesn't proselytize or preach, she said. It doesn't have missionaries. In fact, the thought of such is distasteful to a Wiccan. One just knew "deep in your gut" if Wicca was for him or her. "We are a quiet bunch and prefer to work our magick behind the scenes and in ways to help, not hinder or harm. There are bad folk who say they are Wiccan or witches but they are not. The Goddess simply will not work with anyone whose only intention is to harm or force another being. There are forces that can be harnessed by those with ill intent but the price for using them is incredibly high and they stand out like a sore thumb to anyone with any sensitivity. . . . This is why I don't speak often about my beliefs because so many media images make it sound silly or weird. Wicca teaches that there is no one way or only way to find truth or know the Godhead. If a person lives sincerely and their intention is to commune with the Powers that BE and they practice what they preach then we are all on the same pathway just different flavors so to speak. Tolerance is fundamental to Wicca."

. . . . .

I had felt the stillness of God as I'd read Angela's words. I don't mean that I'd been tempted to forsake Jesus and become Wiccan. I think it was more of a God-given mutual respect. I appreciated the way Angela had explained her beliefs to me in a calm, nonjudgmental way. She'd given me peace.

But that peace had been as I'd sat alone in my office reading her email.

Ten days later, I sat alone outside a bookstore, my right knee frenetically bouncing as I waited to interview them. In my ignorance of Wicca, I wondered if Angela would be wearing black and purple and satanic symbols. But shockingly, instinctively, I recognized them as they walked toward me. They looked like any other mall-shopping, suburban twosome.

Kai was an average height, average weight twenty-five-year-old in long, baggy shorts. His frizzy brown hair was pulled into a ponytail that hung down the middle of his back. I could picture his fingers rapidly moving a game stick. In fact, Kai did spend every Saturday afternoon playing Dungeons & Dragons.

Angela was a short, pale, and lumpy fifty-year-old wearing jeans and a T-shirt. She looked slightly disheveled as if she had too many chores to do. "Oh, hush," she scolded Kai as they walked past me and into the store.

I chortled.

Once we sat down together, Angela quickly began talking while Kai sat listening. They were the opposite in email. With the exception of Angela's words about Wicca, she typed brief notes and said she'd write more but never did. Kai wrote lengthy letters, including one where he explained that they'd met through Alt.com, ten months before. They'd emailed each other, then talked on the phone a few times, and finally met at a restaurant near Angela's home. Kai was immediately taken with Angela's looks.

She has short red hair, green eyes, and, as Kai had described, is a big, beautiful woman. "I tend to find myself attracted to bigger women," he'd written. "But then again, I don't really look for just one quality in a woman (as in breasts, butt, legs, etc.) to find her attractive. I tend to look at the whole person. I'm not going to turn down or rule out a playmate just because she has no tits, or she's too short, or too skinny."

Angela and Kai intended to have a one-weekend romp. Six months later, they were living together, pursuing the BDSM life together and, eventually, swinging, too, because Angela likes a variety of partners. "This is not to say that she is a bed-hopper," Kai had defended. "The partners she continues to see, she has a connection with and is friends with them. And I'm ok with that."

The smoggy spring day that I interviewed them, Angela told me she was already involved in swinging—thanks to a lover she'd had between her first and second marriages—and was dabbling on the edges of kink, too—spanking—when a full-blown desire for kink emerged, thanks to a man she met on AFF, just a year ago. "At least when I'm in the old folks home, I'll have some interesting stories," she laughed.

Angela described herself as a person who takes chances, as long as she feels reasonably safe. After all, she pointed out, pain and pleasure are very close kin, and with either, a person experiences an adrenaline rush. Though the "giving over" in kink is pleasurable, Angela said, she enjoys more the dominant role. "I definitely have a sadistic side. I get pleasure from giving consensual pain."

Oh, Lord, that reminded me of Al. But unlike Al, I thought Angela must be a tenderhearted sadist. She began warning me, protecting me, as our conversation moved to swinging, offering to take me to a local on-premise swing club so that I'd be safe. Apparently, it was the dive bar of swing clubs. The cost was just $30 per couple. There was no screening of patrons. "If you have a pulse, are upright, and have money, you can get in." And like most swing clubs, it was "bring your own bottle."

"Don't drink when you're there," she cautioned me. "You need to keep your wits about you." When three or more people are together sexually, there is so much stimulation that it feeds off itself. That arousal combined with alcohol could result in people tossing out all rules and manners. "A single female needs to watch her back."

I laughed, though it was probably nervously, as Angela made clear that she meant her statement both figuratively and literally.

"The mood can change quickly. It can be dead as a doornail for one and a half hours, and then sex is happening."

The fantasy, she said, is wonderful. "The reality is scary, though, because you become dehumanized. Emotions are put on the back burner."

Then she began caretaking me again. "It's okay to sublimate on occasion, but use caution and common sense." Someone can request an invitation into sex simply by making eye contact or touching a potential partner on a non-sexual area of the body. And as Angela emphasized to me that a single woman simply observing at a swing club can be taken advantage of no matter how assertive she is, I stared into her green eyes behind pink-lensed glasses. I studied the pastel threads in the tiny flowers embroidered around the scooped neckline of her green T-shirt. On one wrist she wore a large watch; on the other she wore a black leather and silver chain bracelet.

My gaze moved back to Angela's neck, and I asked her about the necklace she wore. It depicted three circles. The lone circle at the top represented a Dominant, she said. The two circles below it represented a submissive and a switch. Angela wore the necklace all the time, including at work, where she was a nurse taking care of emotionally and mentally challenged children. Many of her coworkers knew she was into kink. They didn't know about her swing side. "Kink is more accepted," she said.

• • • • •

In their private kink play, Angela and Kai were both switches—constantly revolving between Dominant and submissive so quickly that they could rotate roles as fast as eight times in one minute, all by reading the body language that flows between them.

I found myself curious to watch and see how that worked, wondering if I could detect the role changes in their bodies and faces. But I didn't exactly confess that to them. While they may have been comfortable in being observed, I still wasn't so sure I'd be comfortable in observing. They flog, discipline, spank, play with knives, torture breasts, and practice abrasion play, which can involve smoothing rabbit hair gloves embedded with tacks across the skin.

Finally, Kai began to speak, as if he was getting ever so slightly comfortable with me. I took that as a compliment. I knew from his emails that he was a shy man who, since childhood, had struggled with stuttering. And like Sadistic Bastard, as well as Al, a former girlfriend had introduced him to the Lifestyle. She liked him to pull her by the hair and hold a knife to her throat. "She was scared and wet." Kai liked it, too.

I watched his brown eyes as he spoke.

Maybe he liked it because he isn't a mean or angry man, he said, though he admitted he doesn't vent his feelings. Rather, he releases them through kink play. Kai "joneses," he said, over bondage be it with tape, chain, or rope.

Angela then boasted that she could hold someone in place with her mind.

"If we can synchronize our breathing, stay close to each other, and I can provide sufficiently potent sensations, then I can restrain or hold that person in place by my mind/my control without the physical use of restraints. It's like a snake swaying and holding the attention of a bird."

More obviously, she knows whenever something is going wrong for Kai, because he begins to stutter. She gently calms him by simply placing her hand on his leg.

Just as I suspected, Angela admitted she was tenderhearted, but then she voiced again that she has a sadistic side. "Because of that," she said, "I have to keep a tight monitor on myself." I stared at the sweet pink lipstick on her lips as she said that and as she added that she prefers humiliating people to controlling them. "I can constantly feel in conflict with myself or I can have a way to channel this."

· · · · ·

I thought about her words as I climbed into bed that night with leftover Chinese food and Krispy Kreme doughnuts. Angela had told me she believes she's "damn sexy," despite being roly-poly.

"It doesn't mean I can't tear up photos of myself," she'd said while admitting her road to damn sexy self-confidence had been a "progressive thing." "If you look available, you look sexy," she'd said. "If you gather up courage to do it the first time, you'll get some reinforcement."

I wanted such confidence.

· · · · ·

Maybe that's why I'm racing over to the east side of Austin, searching for Angela and SAADE. Or maybe it's because psychology has always fascinated me, and a seminar on the psychology of bondage sounds interesting. I see SAADE, on a corner, in an AIDS services office, with a black iron gate around the parking lot, just as Angela described. "We will be looking for you," she emailed me, ". . . not going to leave you all alone with a bunch of kinky strangers." Still, I'm angst-ridden as I swing into the parking lot—Angela told me there would be practical demonstrations and, possibly, nudity. "lol," she said. I wasn't so sure.

With the exception of one empty handicap space, the parking lot is filled with cars and people. People with long hair, people with

short hair, people dressed in black, and people smoking. I swerve
back onto the street and around the corner to park on a side street.
Then I rush up to the front door to see Kai waiting for me. He's
looking sparkling clean and shyly boyish despite the thinning hair
on his young head. He starts to open the door for me, then thinks,
and enters before me.

I follow him into an office packed with kinksters. I spot Angela
in the crowd. She has freshly washed and styled hair, is wearing a
short black skirt, red blouse, and little black booties that come just
to her ankles, revealing her white, fleshy legs. She holds a clear plastic container of grocery store bakery cookies—refreshments for the
group—and tells me I must sign a waiver with Trinity, a redheaded
grandmotherly type who's belting out her fondness for BDSM.

Before I make my way up to Trinity, and the basket of brightly
colored condoms on top of the desk that she sits behind, I hear, "Do
you remember me?" I glance around and see a tall woman with
short, black hair curled into finger-sized ringlets. She's a friend from
my past, a former Realtor and Girl Scout leader. I give her a big
hug. I can't tell if she's surprised to see me, but I'm definitely not
surprised to see her. We'd drifted in different directions just as she
started getting into the Lifestyle. More truthfully, I drifted away.
I was uncomfortable the last time I was in her home. It felt filled
with black vibes from bondage and domination. I was especially
uncomfortable knowing that she was rearing children in that environment.

As I stand in the AIDS services office, my past fears and anxie-
ties are replaced with relief and gratitude to see someone I know
and trust—and to see her dressed just as I remember her, in a nondescript shift, and carrying her ever-present bottle of water. I wonder if her house keys are snapped onto a hook inside her purse so
that she always knows where to find them, just as they'd been when
we'd spent time together.

But I move on to Trinity, whose elderly looks—at least to me—
don't seem in sync with her lifestyle. I sign the waiver without

reading it, figuring I'm signing away my life, then fork over five dollars and show my driver's license for ID.

Moments later, I find myself watching a hefty middle-aged woman who's caught my attention because she appears to be in such a bad mood. Her hair is dyed black. Her nose is pierced. And she wears a black skirt and a black see-through blouse. I can't stop staring at her black bra and the large mole on the middle of her back. Now she's demanding time to smoke. *Uh-oh.* She seems like a tough one. Then I discover she's Lady Gwendolyn, the very same woman Angela told me I needed to talk to before entering the seminar. Lady Gwendolyn asks if I mind her cigarette smoke. I lie and tell her I can handle it. Calmed by the nicotine, she's kind and likable. After she tells me I can't tape record the seminar but can take notes, I walk down the corridor to enter the classroom.

It's a long, narrow, hot room crammed with people sitting in chairs, sitting on the floor, and standing against the walls. Lady Gwendolyn opens the seminar by introducing me, warning the SAADE membership of my presence. Most of the members take it in stride, but one woman, standing next to Lady Gwendolyn, erupts with shock and anger. Why wasn't she told about this before? she wants to know. She's Lady Sapphire, the presenter of the night's talk. She's another senior citizen with dyed red hair. Dyed red hair and gray hair seem to be the dominant colors in the room. Lady Sapphire says she fears I will steal her copyrighted material.

Lady Gwendolyn explains that she only found out about my attendance the night before. She turns to the audience and asks if anyone objects to my presence. No one raises a hand. A middle-aged woman with a shaved head holds Lady Sapphire to comfort her. "I promise I won't steal your material," I say. I put away my pad and pen as a show of good faith. My friend from my past vouches for my integrity. I'm thankful for her kindness, but Lady Sapphire isn't appeased.

Lady Gwendolyn offers to type up an agreement in which I swear not to steal Lady Sapphire's material. Lady Sapphire finally agrees to that. She then brings out rope and begins binding members' hands with what she calls Texas handcuffs.

"What about the author?" someone shouts from the back of the room. I have absolutely no desire to be bound, especially not by Lady Sapphire. I look her over. Though her hair is cut in a bit of a Dorothy Hamill do from 1976, Lady Sapphire's demeanor is pure rural. Her eyeglasses look like one-hour wire frames. Her inexpensive, muted-green-print, sleeveless dress reveals white, scarred, toneless arms. Its neckline is slightly scooped but fully covers her breasts, which are aligned with her protruding stomach. The dress is also shapeless and doesn't stop until it reaches her ankles. Slump-shouldered, Lady Sapphire looks like she's about to go grocery shopping on a hot summer day.

I lift up my hands to her, as I feel the call from the back of the room is a double-dog dare, and I have to prove that I can go along with this group. Sitting cross-legged on the floor, my hands stretched above my head and pointing toward Lady Sapphire's belly, I feel like I look like a supplicant. I don't like that, but I keep a smile on my face.

"S S C . . . Safe, sane, and consensual," Lady Sapphire says. She looks down at me, the rope stretched taut between her hands. "I don't believe in that."

As she states that she believes in adding an R for risks, for knowing the risks, I nod my head and zone out, thinking about Lord Master Dominant Patrick, my Sadistic Bastard. There's nothing safe and sane about BDSM, he said. If anyone dies during this, there certainly will be a guilty verdict.

Lady Sapphire handcuffs me with the rope.

I place my bound hands in my lap trying to find a comfortable position for them. The rope's loose enough that I can probably push the ends with my thumbs and break myself free. But I'm afraid that Lady Sapphire will catch me, that the group won't like me. Every time I glance around, someone's watching me. I finally succumb to my state and listen to the talk Lady Sapphire so feared I'd steal.

She speaks about bondage for people who like to hug, bondage for people who are claustrophobic, bondage that creates enticing photographs but can kill if a person is left hanging for more than a few seconds. The crowd laughs. The humor escapes me.

I want to know what makes a person *want* to be tied up.

Lady Sapphire says that if a person can't stand to be blindfolded, have them put their hands behind their neck, bind their hands, then push their arms together and bind their elbows. This, she says, has the same effect as a blindfold—the submissive can't see what's being done to his body. She bends to show us how she can't see her body.

I squirm on the floor.

"Are you okay?" Angela says, her voice concerned.

"Yes. It's just that my legs are cramping."

Eventually, Lady Sapphire begins to move around the room, asking people what they're feeling before untying them. One wants to be tied tighter. A few have already untied themselves. She stands above me and looks down. "What are you feeling?"

"Anger."

"Oh," she laughs to the crowd, "I love emotion. Anger at me?"

"I thought this was supposed to be about trust. But tying my hands so that I can't take notes, when I'd already closed up my pad and put away my pen, shows that you don't trust me."

Lady Sapphire unties me. "What are you feeling now?"

"Boredom."

"Oh," she chuckles. "We've gone from anger to boredom."

But I truly am bored. I haven't seen or heard one interesting thing. Certainly no nudity. And by now I'm thinking I want nudity. But most of all, I haven't gotten an inkling of an answer as to why people want to be bound. And this lecture was supposed to be on the psychology of bondage. Obviously, Lady Sapphire's definition of psychology is very different from mine.

As she begins to move away, she says to me, "This will teach you to bring a tape recorder."

"I have one," I respond. "It's in my purse, but I was asked before-hand not to use it. I do what I'm told."

I think Lady Sapphire will like my words because I think she's a Dominant, but she walks away without a smile. She later confesses to the group that despite her name she's a submissive.

. . . . .

With my hands freed, though, I'm able to look around the room. I see that Angela's left wrist is tied loosely with white string to Kai's right wrist. She whispers to me that she can handle being bound only because she's tied to Kai and because her right hand is free. She shakes her free hand. "I'm claustrophobic," she says.

I understand. To some degree, I am, too. But my rope had been loose, and I knew my legs were free to stand and run.

I look behind me. I see two, tall, enviably skinny, fashionably dressed, gorgeous women—one dark-haired, one bleached blond and tattooed—sitting on the floor. Each leans blissfully against a knee of the Dominant they share. To my left, more women with the trademark chain and small silver padlock around their necks sit peacefully at the feet of their Dominants. They remind me of pup-pies happy to be sleeping on their masters' shoes.

I make brief eye contact with others watching me before my attention is swayed to a woman speaking to Lady Sapphire. It's not her words that grab me. It's her tone. She sounds stoned. Yes, she says dreamily, the bondage worked on her—she's transformed. Like a drug, it's made her high. The room erupts into applause thanking Lady Sapphire for her seminar.

I grab a handout, thank Angela and Kai, race out of the room and to my car. I'm exhausted. I can't believe I gave in and let myself be bound. My tires nearly squeal as I U-turn to get out of there.

At home, I glance down at Lady Sapphire's handout and laugh out loud. "Copyright 1993 Michael Nelson," it says. No wonder she feared I'd use "her" copyrighted material.

I stand, clasp my hands around the back of my neck, and hold my elbows together in front of me, just as Lady Sapphire suggested binding someone who can't wear a blindfold. I bend and twist to see if I can see what's going on around my body, if I could see someone striking me, as Lady Sapphire said I couldn't. I can see everything.

"Obviously, I'm not bondage material," I emailed a friend. "I must admit other sexual desires are rising, ones that I wish I didn't have because shrinks tell me they are so unhealthy. Oh, well, thinking and acting are two different things. And I don't even have the opportunity to act."

Chapter 21

. . . . .

Like Coyote, all I thought about was sex. Then again, how could one spend every day talking to people about the most intimate details of their sex lives and not have desires of one's own arise? "It's just an amazing world out there," I wrote Rose. "If I could just find someone I'm attracted to . . ."

But just as I couldn't finish my sentence for Rose, I felt I must keep those desires hidden deep within me. Besides, I had my sex freaks to reveal secrets, and since I was living vicariously through them, I checked in with Jessica.

She'd been with Ryan again—the Catholic schoolteacher—and he'd asked her what she wanted in a relationship. She called that "perhaps the most loaded question in the history of creation." Still, she answered him. She wanted great sex. She wanted to be held. She wanted to be told she was beautiful. She wanted great conversation, to be challenged, to be kept on edge, to be excited every time she saw him. "I want to want you so bad that when I see you my brain starts reeling." She went on for at least thirty-nine wants, sometimes with multiple wants in one sentence, but the one thing

Jessica didn't mention to Ryan was kisses. And the one thing she dwelled on to me was that she desperately wanted kisses.

"granted, i think learning how to kiss someone new takes time, as everyone has their own style. but with these guys, perhaps because it isn't a relationship, perhaps because we haven't been together all that many times, it just hasn't been a priority. kissing is so intimate, even more so in my book, than having sex. maybe that's it as well— these are not situations that allow for intimacy."

Intimacy. That word made me shudder. How in the world was I going to continue to live vicariously through Jessica if she kept seeking intimacy?

But the very next thing she typed was "wynn."

Thank God.

"wynn is a skinny, very pretty, very shy, very fucking smart, 25-year-old, who i met up with last week. liberal as hell, vegan, very much up my alley." But she was having a hard time picturing him as a sexual creature, even though they were planning on meeting for sex—"i suppose." The "i suppose" was because Wynn was still living with his ex-girlfriend. But it was also because Jessica knew she'd have to make the first move, and that's not what she wanted. She wanted to be "taken by storm." She also fretted that she wasn't smart enough for Wynn.

And with that one email, I finally realized why I was so enamored with this twenty-five-year-old, sexually liberated chef whom I thought I had absolutely nothing in common with—she and I had *so* much in common. We were both so fucking insecure and yet so self-confident. And we were both confused as heck.

A couple of days later, Jessica sat in her apartment writing me, anxiously killing time, waiting for Wynn to phone, to see if he was going to come over. She glanced at the clock on her computer. He was supposed to phone around 10:30 P.M. "i'm actually quite curious as to how this dude is in bed. he wrote such shamelessly hot pornography i could hardly stand it. . . . i keep thinking that if any of what he writes translates into the bedroom then i'm golden.

i imagine him to be a very sensitive lover. that could have its pluses, after having my ass reamed two weeks ago by ralph."

The phone rang. Wynn was on his way.

"i'm sorry, you're just going to have to bear with me and my rambling incoherent thoughts until he gets here. for all the self-confidence i exude, or pretend to exude, i am not well-versed in this arena, whatever that might be. the arena of sex with essentially a stranger who i could potentially, more realistically than any of the other dudes i've met, really like, as our thoughts and wavelengths are so similar. for that reason alone, because i see some potential, a part of me wonders if i should hold out. but i don't even know what he wants, what he's looking for."

When she'd asked him what he was doing on Craigslist, he'd said he was lonely. "that reminds me of 65 year old men. not 25 year olds," she said. But then she admitted, "perhaps it's easier to have sex with a total stranger than actually pursue something."

Yes.

"i cannot get over suzy the fact that i posted this ad, this fucking blasé, call me, we'll talk and fuck ad, and now feel compelled, for strange men, to live up to it. not with all of them, obviously, as i've not had sex with more than i have had sex with. but why? why why why? because on paper, i can say anything, be anyone, and when i have to live up to or follow through with it, i lose some of the ballsi-ness that got me there in the first place."

Just as she'd told me after she'd been with Ralph, she stated that what she really sought was the buildup. That was enough—because "the end result can often be disappointing. i suppose this is life."

The buildup. I'm not sure I've ever experienced the buildup. I don't remember ever breathlessly waiting for some guy to arrive. Am I that uncaring? That cold? More likely I think I've given up. Since first grade, when I first lusted over a gorgeous dark-haired boy named Travis, I prayed to Jesus for a boyfriend. I never got one. The closest I ever came was a couple of briefly consummated asso-ciations with married men.

Oh, wait, I do remember one time eagerly and anxiously waiting for a man to arrive at my apartment. But maybe that's because moments before he knocked on my door, spinach stems blasted up and out of my garbage disposal, past the sink and onto the ceiling. Their green juice rained from my cream-colored ceiling and onto my silk blouse. So when I opened my door, I'm not sure I was breathless for him or because of the dripping spinach.

Of course, he was married.

That night, Jessica and Wynn talked about politics and the state of the world, and she smiled, thinking they were so on the same wavelength. Then she got up to go the bathroom, glanced over at her computer and noticed the time. 2 A.M. They'd been talking for three hours. She turned to Wynn. She gulped. "Well, if we're going to do something about this, then let's do it now. But if you have to leave, it's fine. I understand."

He walked over to her. "I'm staying."

They stood in the doorway. They hemmed and hawed. Finally, she forced herself to utter, "Let's go to the bedroom, as this is where these things happen."

"then we were off and running," she wrote.

"good god. there was some fucking passion behind it, some drive beyond just having an orgasm. hands interwoven in hair, fingers running up and down bodies, on faces, touching like how i want to be touched. with interest and regard and respect. it was so nice. it was beyond nice. it reminded me of the first time my girlfriend and i got together.

"we didn't have intercourse (too much pressure can sometime equal lack of an erection, making sex difficult, as i am learning) but ran the gamut of other activities for well over two hours. at one point, when he was straddling me and i was on my back, i asked him what he wanted me to do, or simply what he wanted in general. he said, 'i just want to taste you.' ohmigod. i melted into a puddle in the bed. it was so hot."

She invited him to spend the night.

The next morning, she walked him to the door. They hemmed, hawed, and smiled again, not knowing what to say or do.

"I hope we can get together again soon," Jessica eventually muttered. Then she said what she always said after sex. "Thank you." She kissed him on the cheek, kissed him on the mouth, and went about her day, though she found herself spacing out at work.

"this is the involvement i want to be having. this is the attachment. . . . he is it."

A day later, Jessica admitted for the first time something I should have picked up on, but in my excitement of living through this twenty-five-year-old woman, I hadn't. Jessica was lonely.

And Wynn, she believed, had possibility. "it feels like it could be sustainable in a healthier, happier way. or maybe that's what i wanted from the beginning but was not willing to admit. . . . but maybe, maybe maybe it's too soon to say, maybe maybe maybe i should calm down, but maybe i wouldn't have to compromise anything and maybe that would be really really nice."

Chapter 22

. . . . .

Maybe. Maybe. Maybe.

Jessica's maybes stuck in my brain. As did her loneliness. While her loneliness had her creating mildly insane drama via Craigslist, mine had me writing a book about sex in the hope that I could work through my own sexual issues and find a date. Okay, maybe that's not really true. Maybe I didn't want a date. Maybe I just wanted a lover. No, that's not true either, because a lover sounds like a relationship. I want a friend with whom, on occasion—rare occasion— I can have dinner, conversation, and sex . . . and then we go our separate ways.

Is that a lover or a fuck buddy? But wasn't I in therapy to try to learn how to do relationships? To learn why sexual relationships scare the hell out of me? Relationships, particularly sexual ones, involve emotional intimacy . . . or at least they're supposed to. At least that's what I'd been taught growing up, and I wanted to believe that was true. But I don't trust men enough to be emotionally intimate with them. And I don't know why men terrify me so. They just do. God, they do.

• • • • •

Rex emailed me that he'd had phone sex with two new women, both wanting daddy/daughter play. *Oh, God*. The mere mention of such makes something putrid rise in my throat and nearly lodge there, before I force it back down. I forced it back down because I had to do my job. I asked Rex what he said during such.

"I just improvise differently each time. Wanna listen in? LOL."

No, I didn't. "Yeah," I answered, "I do wish I could listen in and take notes. That's what this book is about."

But Rex didn't think most women would go for me listening in, if they knew about it. "But if I didn't tell them and you just were quiet, I would do that for you."

There was another obstacle, though. Rex never knew when he was going to have phone sex. It was always spur of the moment, whenever he and one of his friends happened to be online at the same time, ". . . or if I happen to meet someone in a chat room who is willing."

Rex said he frequented daddy/daughter role-playing chat rooms because there were more women in them.

Ugh. I couldn't imagine.

• • • • •

The next day, I received an email from Rex that included a daddy/daughter story he'd written for a woman he'd met on AFF before he'd married his current wife. Back then, he and the woman had met in a parking lot, where they'd sat in her car, kissed and groped each other, until she said she wanted to masturbate while she watched him do the same. "I came all over her dashboard and she came hard and loud watching me."

That I found rather interesting—the coming all over the dashboard. But as I read farther down his email, to his daddy/daughter story, I couldn't handle it anymore, especially when he talked about

"Mom" and the daddy convincing the daughter that her mother was fucking another man, as if that made the dad's incest okay. The story printed out to two single-spaced pages. I could only read a few words per paragraph. It disgusted me. It sickened me. And I could not fathom how—why—that turned a woman on. Had she been abused? Is that why? Is that the only way she could find emotional intimacy with her father? To imagine having sex with him? Or had she not been abused and that's why the fantasy didn't seem sick, violent . . . the ultimate betrayal?

Yes, I know I'm being judgmental. But through my true crime books and my friends, I've seen the damage done by fathers, stepfathers, and father figures who have sex with their children.

That didn't dissuade me, though, from giving Rex my phone number when he notified me that he'd set up a phone sex session for two days later so that I could listen. After all, as I said before, this was my job, and Rex needed my number to dial me into the call, which unbeknownst to his sex partner would be a three-way. Then, without me inquiring, he pointed out that this sex partner wasn't into the daddy/daughter thing.

Thank God.

· · · · ·

It's a Monday in May, and I sit in my home, at my desk, my wire-rim glasses perched on the tip of my nose. I grab a pen and yellow legal pad and click on my tape recorder. Via a three-way conference call, I eavesdrop on Rex as he sits in his home and has phone sex with a married woman in El Paso, Texas, while Rex's wife sits at her job and his stepchildren sit at school.

Rex's voice is low, soft, measured, and sexy. "I walk in with a hard-on. Turn you around. Rub my cock against your ass." He inserts lots of slow cooing ums, ahs, and moans. "Squeeze those big hips. Bite your neck. Lick your ear. I'm making my dick throb against you."

She groans with pleasure.

"I turn you around and grope your big tits." He pinches her nipples. "Mmm, you're making me so big." He pulls off her shorts, pushes them down to her ankles, and grabs her "nice round ass" with his "big hands." "Squeeze it, spank you, ah, spank you with my dick. Spread you open. Ah, yeah." His speech is breathless. "Rub my head up and down your pussy lips, rub your clit with it."

She moans, "Huh?"

"Rub your clit with it," he says louder.

And while I quietly chuckle over her "huh," she groans happily.

"Rub my shaft up and down your clit. Spanking your ass."

"Oh, God," she breathes.

"Oh, yeah," he returns. "That hot pussy juice all over my cock head." He rubs his penis up and down her "swollen cunt lips" and spanks her rear. "Telling you what a filthy whore you are."

"Fuck me quickly," she whispers.

"Is that what you want, baby?" He calls her a slut and her moans get harder. He breathes like he's rubbing himself. "Wish you were my neighbor."

"I'd be fucking ready," she responds.

He says he watched her house to see when her "hubby" leaves for work. As soon as the husband's car turns the corner, Rex would be over. She'd still be in her nightgown. He'd rip it off her, throw her on the bed, climb on top of her, bend down, suck on her tits, and bite her nipples.

"Oooh."

"Squeeze those big juicy tits together and suck on both nipples at the same time. . . . Lick my way down your body until my mouth is on your pussy. Licking your lips. Sucking in all your juice. Spreading you open with my hands. Shoving my tongue inside your pussy. Oh, sucking on your clit."

"Oh, God."

"Flicking it with my tongue." He begins making tongue-flicking sounds. "Rrrrrrr."

She groans.

"Rrrrrrr."

Quickly, I cover my mouth remembering that we're on a three-way connection and she can probably hear the guffaws that are about to burst out of me.

"Rrrrrrr," he repeats, and each time he does, she groans louder, then grunts until she screams with ecstasy. "Yeah, come all over my face baby. Rrrrrr." I feel like I'm listening to a porno movie without the visuals. I'm not sure I'm getting hot, though, because I'm trying so hard not to laugh, as he rrrrrrs off and on for twenty seconds before they begin round two for orgasm number two.

They go through intercourse, complete with animalistic huffing and pumping sound effects. Maybe I'm turned on after all, because I find myself suddenly thirsty. I reach for a glass of water and take a sip, clanking the glass against the phone. Yikes. I know the hard clunk has echoed across the line. But that doesn't stop them. He pumps and huffs in growing intensity and increasing volume for thirty seconds, before she grunts loudly as she comes again, and they move on to oral sex.

"Suck my dick, you cheating married whore."

She begins to make sucking sounds and sucks for well more than a minute while he oh, yeah, oh, yeah, oh, yeahs and finally makes guttural noises like he's about to come. Then he says he's pulling his cock out of her mouth. She seems unhappy about that. So he slaps her with his penis and rubs it on her face.

"Oh, yeah, give it to me," she responds.

"You like sucking your pussy . . ."

"Uh, sucking his cock," she corrects in a whisper, then keeps right on with her slurping and kissing sounds, while I stifle my giggle over her editing. They continue on and on and on, until his timbre grows harsh and berating.

"That's it, you cheap slut. Suck my dick! . . . That's it, you filthy whore. That's it, you cock-sucking slut."

My laughter vanishes.

Her slurps get faster and harder, until she and Rex return to intercourse and more pounding, jamming animal sounds. He pushes harder, breathes harder, and she cries out, "Yeah, yeah, yeah, ooooooh!" But he keeps on pumping. For approximately two minutes, he's inside her, until he finally tells her he's leaning back. "That's it, baby. Like it up the ass, don't you?"

"Fuck you," she softly gasps.

"Oh, yeah. Who's my whore?" He proceeds to anal sex. "Show me what a cock slut you are for my dick."

"Oh, baby," she answers, "I'll be the little whore that you need."

At that, their tones turn gentle and their words tender. I don't understand. What I mean is I don't understand how the hurling of foul insults can cause tenderness between two people. They chitchat as though they're having post-coital pillow talk. Then she whispers, "You can fuck me any way you want me. Bounce me on your cock."

"That's it." Aggression and rage fly into Rex's voice. "Ride my dick, you whore. That's it, buck me! You filthy slut. Come on, you cock-loving whore. Cheating married slut. You big-titted whore."

My stomach feels leaden.

"Fuck. Oh, fuck. . . . Fill my ass with your cum."

"Spread those cheeks open." He shoves inside her. Ooof, oof, oof, and they climax together.

They finish with her performing oral sex on him again. At length he moans softly. And thirty minutes after the phone call started, she says, "That's the first time you've let me make you come twice."

"Um-huh."

Suddenly, I feel like he's been performing for me.

"Bye, baby," he says to her. "You still there?" he says to me.

"Yep," I answer. "So what are you actually doing during all of this?"

"Masturbating."

I offer to let him go clean up.

"You don't want to ask any questions or anything?"

"I think as I'm talking to you I'm turning embarrassed, red-faced."

"Well, you shouldn't be embarrassed. If anybody should be embarrassed it should be me."

"You really enjoy this?" I say.

"It's not better than real sex, but it's certainly different from what I get with my wife."

"How's it different?"

He reminds me that his wife doesn't like French kissing or oral sex—giving or receiving. "Pretty much, when she has an orgasm, she's done. If I didn't come, she feels bad but not bad enough to do anything about it. . . . She was a preacher's daughter. She was a good little girl. And sex is just not a big deal to her."

"But you have a good marriage?"

"Other than that, yeah. . . . We have a lot in common. We laugh and get along great. I've expressed my frustration to her, but," he sighs, "it doesn't seem to do any good."

"So you think you'll stick with your marriage?" They've been married for less than six years.

"I think so."

"Is there anything else you want to tell me?" To be honest, I'm wanting off the phone. I've been wanting off it ever since they finished having sex. I don't know if I'm spent or discombobulated or just wanting to get away from all of the cock slut, filthy slut, cock-loving whore, cheating married slut, big-titted whore talk. I'm from the era when women marched in the streets to demand that they not be called such. On top of that, that's the very kind of demeaning, hateful, raging talk that has turned me off of men.

But Rex wants to keep talking, so I keep listening as he says, "I still like sex on the nasty/sleazy side. I love taboo sex, which would be the best way to put it."

I guess I don't. I guess I'm more like my mother's friend than I thought—I want sweet sex. Then again, when it comes right down to the facts of the heart and the brain, it's not just a relationship that terrifies me. Having sex scares me, too. So as much as I say I want to have sex, I'm not sure I could actually *do* it. Oh, God, I'm confused.

Chapter 23

. . . . .

"Suzy, I know you are supposed to be the one asking all the questions," Coyote wrote, "but I am dying to know how you can talk about all this sexual stuff with different people, without becoming a little turned on or worked up yourself? There is no way I could do it without wanting to join in or at least watch and see for myself—LOL. And then I would probably be masturbating for sure."

My fingers lay motionless on the keyboard.

Six minutes later, I finally typed, "I'm gonna wait to answer your questions. My mother is on her way over to my house, and it does make me feel a bit freaky to be doing all this sex research with her around."

In fact, not just my family made me feel freaky about my sex research. I'd made the mistake of telling a friend about my phone sex eavesdropping. By the time I told her, I'd gotten over the cocksucking whore talk and had started giggling again about the sound effects—"rrrrrrrrrr," "ooof, oof, oof"—and the way Rex's partner had corrected him when he'd made mistakes in his descriptions. I had to share my laughter with someone. But my friend didn't find it funny. She found it an intrusion on the woman's privacy. She said she couldn't hear anymore.

So now part of me feels like a pervert and part of me is angry at my friend for being so quick to judge. She considers herself so liberal and sexually progressive, but she's never done phone sex. She's never even kissed a woman.

Consequently, when Coyote asked if I was getting turned on, I didn't know what I was feeling. I do know that by the next day, reality was hitting me. I was growing tired of hearing everyone cheat. But I also kept thinking about Rex and how his tele-partner had said that was the first time he'd let her bring him to orgasm more than once. I was curious about that, and I asked him about it.

Usually he came just once during phone sex, he said. "But it had been a while since I had had an orgasm, so I was still hard after cumming and had kept stroking my cock because I could tell she was still horny. So I came again."

A half hour later, he called her a second time because he knew she'd still be horny and he wanted more. At first, Rex simply told me that he "fucked her again and came again, too." Eventually, he provided details: "The scenario that I used brought you into it. Not you personally, but a neighbor who had come over to visit her, spied on us while we fucked, and we caught her doing so. I then had her bring you into the room and we both had sex with you. It was a scenario that she never gets tired of. Although she likes it when there are two men using her, she really gets off watching me fuck someone else, as long as I save my cum for her."

There was more.

"It was a huge turn-on for me to know you were listening. Like having someone peek in the door at you while you are having sex with someone. That was another reason I kept stroking my cock after I came the first time. And I will also admit that even while I was chatting with you, I was still stroking my cock and had gotten hard again."

I would have never dreamed he was doing that. I was a bit freaked, a bit offended, and a bit honored. But lordy mercy, I'd never admit that last one to my friend, my shrink . . . or Coyote. Coyote was just too close. We'd sat across from each other and looked into each other's face. Rex and I hadn't done that. He hadn't even hinted at wanting such. That made him still safe.

Safe.

That seemed to be a word that came up a lot during my research. For me and for my sex freaks.

· · · · ·

Robin remembers the day specifically. It was a Saturday of a multiweek business trip to London. After decades of hiding bras, girdles, and panties under her men's clothing and wearing women's blouses and pants that didn't look too feminine, Robin waited in an upstairs sitting room of a full-service cross-dressing shoppe. She was excited . . . and she yearned to talk to another cross-dresser. She turned to the woman sitting near her, a woman who was in the process of getting her own cross-dressing makeover. But as Robin tried to start a conversation, all the woman would say was "yes." Robin sipped her tea, before trying again, dying to know how the woman felt about being there. "No," the woman answered, as if she were too overwhelmed to speak.

With that, Robin quietly drank her tea, until a genetically born female came and got her and ushered her to the sales floor. The woman built up Robin's confidence and made her feel pampered. Robin slipped on hips and swayed with them to get their feel. She put on breasts, felt them, and moved with them. She smoothed her hands over the corset and admired her figure. She put on the wig, the makeup, and she looked in the mirror. Her long eyelashes, the very ones that had gotten her ridiculed as a boy, were lush and beautiful. Robin smiled. She felt calm. She felt complete. She thought she looked like her mother.

· · · · ·

Robin was a six-foot-three, fifty-four-year-old, married father of two, mathematician, and cross-dresser from Washington, D.C. She and I had been emailing for a month or more after meeting through Alt.com. We'd spent much of that time communicating about girdles. Robin was obsessed with them, specifically those from the 1940s and 1950s, the kind that every woman from Marilyn Monroe to Barbara Stanwyck had worn in their movies—and my mother had worn to church and even to drink coffee at the homes of her friends.

In fact, I'd worn a tight, white one in junior high to hold up my hose in the days before panty hose existed. Thinking back now, it seemed more like a chastity belt than a girdle. But Robin, who is known as Rob in public and to his family, wants to wear those highly structured, confining girdles today. She can't understand why her wife doesn't love to wear them, too.

Rob's girdle desire began in second grade. He was a self-conscious, unhappy child, who frequently got beaten by the school-yard bullies because he was overweight. He knew a girdle would make him look slimmer, so he pulled on a Platex rubber one, which Robin referred to as "the most sensuous girdle of all." Rob then rolled on support stockings, attached them to the girdle, and left for school. "There was a certain excitement about wearing it and not getting caught."

When Rob was eight years old, his parents discovered his girdle, took it away, and ordered him to stay in his room until he told them why he had it. He wrote his mother a note simply saying he wanted to wear it. He wrote her because his family "was very bad" at discussing feelings.

For the next three years, Rob got better at sneaking his mother's girdles and hiding the ones he'd snatched from the trash after she'd tossed them out. When he was eleven, he suffered a ruptured appendix and had a legitimate excuse to wear a girdle. His aunt, who worked in a corset shop, sent him one.

"So, I got what I wanted, to wear a girdle 24/7. The one I got was an open bottom, so it was not particularly comfortable. A long leg panty girdle is much more comfortable for me."

For some reason that line, that information—"a long leg panty girdle"—seemed too intimate for me, like I finally knew too much. That didn't stop me, though, from reading on.

". . . I was simply too shy to ask for a different style. Whether my mom would have taken me to the corset shoppe for a fitting is unknown. Reading about the fitting for a first girdle is very interesting to me. It's a rite of passage that a girl got in the very old days. They have no such rite today. I guess they all have a first period, but that special rite, along with all the fussing is not done."

I don't recall such a rite of passage or a fitting, though I remember my mother bought that uncomfortable white girdle at Clark-Ayres department store, as I stood next to her, in the back of the store, staring at my feet on the oak wood floors.

Through Rob's teenaged years, he continued "borrowing" his mother's clothing, cross-dressing about once a week when his parents went out for the evening. Around age fifteen, he got caught again. That time, he was sent to a psychiatrist.

"I recall hearing 'queer' from my father. I suppose it was aimed at me, but he'd never say that directly, only indirectly. Looking back, there were lots of serious issues on both sides of the family. Two alcoholic grandfathers. Mom's dad died very young, and my grandmother raised 4 kids on welfare. Father's dad lost big money in the depression and never recovered from it."

Robin expressed sympathy for her father, wondering how he didn't break from the stress.

"What, if anything, rubbed off on me is not fully understood. . . . Perhaps my cross-dressing was crying out for attention. . . . I know that being a kid was no fun for me."

I had to stop and absorb everything that Robin had written me. Maybe that's because I was being inundated with cross-dressing information. Dusty was emailing me the details of his enema play, specifically describing his brand-new silky, navy blue French-cut panties, matching lace bra and garter belt, and black nylon stockings. And Jessica was emailing me that she was "smitten beyond smitten" with Wynn, who'd just come out to her as gender queer, which "means about twelve million things to ten million people."

My perception of "gender queer" equated to the concept of gender fluidity, which, to me, meant psychologically flowing from one gender to the other depending on how one felt that day, that hour, that moment. If one were feeling more male, one might dress, behave, walk and talk more male. If one were feeling more female, one's dress, behavior, walk, and talk might reflect that. Or, one could be both at the same time.

On second thought, maybe I shouldn't have been taken aback that Jessica—a woman who'd just ended a long-term relationship with a woman—would be smitten with a male who considered himself gender queer.

When Jessica asked Wynn what he meant by gender queer, "he said that he's never really felt comfortable with the male paradigm and what society markets to men." He'd changed his name from Jake to Wynn because Wynn was sexually ambiguous. Jessica then asked Wynn if he wanted to have sex with men. "No." She asked him if he wanted to dress in women's clothing. "Maybe sometimes."

He said that all of this was the result of his ex-girlfriend. "She told him that there was an incident two years prior in which she felt that he sexually assaulted her. whoa whoa."

For the two hours after Wynn told Jessica that, they had "hot sweaty, ahh, the best" sex.

As you've heard me say too many times, I couldn't imagine. I'm sorry, but if a woman felt like someone I was dating had sexually assaulted her, and I knew about that, I wouldn't want to date him. Then again, despite the fact that Mr.-Do-You-Have-a-Place-Where-I-Can-Stick-This penis man had attempted to force me into having sex with him, I've shared drinks and meals with him several times throughout the decades since. So I guess I'm not just judgmental, I'm a hypocrite, too.

Besides, I'd never communicated with Wynn. Maybe if I had, maybe I would have discovered that he was a sweet soul.

I'd communicated extensively with Dusty and I liked him. And after I processed everything that Robin had told me, I thanked her for sharing her heart with me.

But I still didn't want to share with Coyote my answer to his question about whether I got turned on by my research. In fact, I didn't answer it.

Instead, he told me he'd been with eleven couples he'd met over the Internet, some couples more than once. Out of those eleven, seven of the husbands had been bisexual. And out of those eleven couples, he'd had additional on-the-sly meetings with two of the wives. On top of that, he'd been with fifteen men he'd met through the Internet, most of whom were married bisexuals. Half of those he'd been with more than once. He'd seen one of them more than a half dozen times and another, who was a cross-dresser, three times. "Looks damn good all dressed up, lol, and can suck you like you wouldn't believe. Will probably see him more too."

Coyote wanted to meet with me to tell me more details in person. And he persisted in asking me if I got turned on by my research. "I'm not asking you to embarrass you. I just want to know. If you want me to mind my own business, just tell me."

I wanted him to mind his own business. Instead, I said, "You know, it's just my job. I guess I think of it like a straight male gynecologist. When he does an exam on a woman, he's really interested but he doesn't get excited. He saves that for his off time with someone special. So, yes, I hang on every word someone tells me. I'm totally fascinated. But it's my job."

And I couldn't meet him again right then, because on the day he had a VA hospital excuse, I had a meeting with a Dominatrix. Then I turned off my computer, climbed into bed, and turned on the TV. Reruns of *Frasier* were on.

Chapter 24

· · · · ·

Lily Ma'am is just as she described—five feet, seven inches tall, silver hair pulled back in a ponytail, and wearing blue jeans, a green and navy print blouse, and a smile. She sits in a straight-back booth with hard wood seats in a chain steak restaurant not far from my house. And she laughs, a lot and easily and heartily. She's a large woman with soft, even skin, as though she washes every day with ninety-nine and forty-four one-hundredths percent pure free Ivory Soap. And because she seems so safe, so pure, I find myself immediately confessing to her about Coyote's query to me—does my work turn me on?

Eagerly, she responds. "I have lots of people ask me, they say, 'Do you find this sexual?' And I go, 'Well,'" she pauses for dramatic effect, " 'yeah.' And they say, 'Are you getting off?' And I'm saying, 'Well, no, not necessarily, because when I'm involved in this sort of thing and I am the person *doing* this to other people, I'm more interested in their reactions. I'm excited in their reaction, but am I having an orgasm? Well, probably not. You're just too involved in what you're doing and trying to be safe rather than letting yourself go off to some place where you're out of control." She chuckles.

"So in that case," I wonder, "what do you get out of it?"

"I'm not saying it's not exciting to me. I think it's that control, that person is letting you do stuff to them that a normal person in a normal situation wouldn't, and that's kind of a—I don't want to say it's an ego thing, but really it kinda is. It makes you feel really pleased that they trust you enough to put themselves into your hands and let you do things to them that most people would find really bizarre."

I hadn't understood the thrill when Al had talked about controlling someone. But with Lily's explanation, I understand more than I want to admit. It is an ego thing when these people confess to me details of their lives that they've never revealed to another soul. It puffs up my chest and brings a smile to my lips that I want to hide.

"Most people who meet me would never, ever think that I was involved with anything that's wasn't just perfectly normal," Lily says, stirring her iced tea.

"I see you playing bridge," I say.

I know she's a BDSMer who sells Mary Kay cosmetics. In fact, I'd pictured her in a pink Mary Kay Cadillac, its trunk full of whips, chains, and nipple clamps. And sitting in the very middle of those whips, chains, and nipple clamps is her Mary Kay sample box. I'd liked her based on that image alone.

"I was the PTA president at my son's kindergarten school," she says.

She's a married, bisexual mother of three, politically independent, though she leans strongly Republican, who was reared Jehovah's Witness and "currently" considers herself an Episcopalian with pagan interests. Angela had introduced us.

And since Lily mentioned her family, I ask about her husband.

She stretches out, "Ummm. My husband, uh, would prefer that I not discuss with you what he does."

Sir Justin, as he's called in the world of BDSM, is Lily's fourth husband.

She married her first husband—"a Witness boy"—right after

high school because she was "really dying to have sex" and "really thought that was going to be great." When they were dating, though, he didn't seem interested in touching her or kissing her.

"I'm sure he was gay. Of course, that's really frowned on when you're born a Jehovah's Witness. . . ."

And when you're born a Southern Baptist, I could add, but don't.

Their marriage lasted two and a half years. "I rushed right out of that first marriage into another marriage, with somebody ten years older than me, because he liked sex and I was really, really wanting to have that kind of experience." Plus, he had children and had custody of them. She wanted children. Her first husband hadn't.

In turn, her second husband—whom she refers to as the Frito man, because he delivered chips to the convenience store where she worked—was, she says, abusive to her. "You know how people do. They tell you, oh, well, if you hadn't done this then I wouldn't be so mad. Or if you would make sure you would do so and so, then I wouldn't have to be irritated with you, or hold you by your throat in the bathroom, you know, to make my point."

She pauses at length, as though she's thinking about it, seeing it in her mind. Then, as if consciously urging herself to be positive, she chipperly chirps, "Anyway, but I got out of that." But the longer Lily talks about that second marriage, the more she seems to have trouble getting the words out of her mouth, as if the pain still chokes her.

"But then I started having more children and, you know, got busy, and now that sort of stuff doesn't really bother me."

I don't believe her.

"You know, because there's a big difference in being abused and doing something in the Lifestyle where it's a totally consensual thing. I'm—I don't ever feel conflicted about that at all because of the consensuality involved. Because if I'm flogging someone or paddling them or doing something to them, it's always negotiated ahead of time. And I know where their limits are. And know that they're really loving it. So it's not like I'm just jerking them up and doing something mean to them, that they're not wanting. And that's a completely different thing. Completely."

I can comprehend that, but at the same time . . . to me . . . there just seems to be so much in Lily's background that . . . well . . . makes her attraction to BDSM understandable.

When she was four or five years old and sitting on the toilet in her playmate Marnie's house, Marnie reached for her daddy's leather belt, turned to Lily, and instructed her not to pull up her panties. Instead, she told her to come over to her. "I want to show you something." Marnie slipped the leather belt between Lily's legs, so that it touched Lily's bare private parts, and lifted her with it.

"As it pressed against my crotch, there was an exciting feeling that I've never forgotten," Lily emailed me. "[Even now,] when I smell leather, my body responds to it."

When I think of Daddy's leather belt, I remember running down the hallway of my childhood home, my mother chasing me, threatening to whip me with Dead Daddy's belt, then stopping at the doorway to the bathroom, where she always, always broke down in tears, dropped the belt, and swatted me with her hand. I then turned and walked into my bedroom, grinning behind her back that I'd gotten away with something—I'd controlled her rather than she controlling me—and laughing to hide the pain that I'd made her cry.

. . . . .

Lily considers her childhood a contradiction. While her religion taught her chastity and self-control, her imagination was focused on sex, trying to figure out how it "worked." When Lily was "quite young," she toyed with water pressure against her privates. By second grade, she was having "a very fun relationship with the little girl next door." While she was still in elementary school, several high school boys told Lily and another friend of hers that they wanted to play a game with them. "And we ended up underneath their pier-and-beam house with our hands held behind our backs and they 'examined us.' Nothing really invasive or scary. It happened several times."

Lily and her friend talked about it and agreed not to tell anyone, "because we found it very exciting that these older boys (we were 10 & 11) were taking that kind of an interest in us, even though as an adult I know it was completely inappropriate, I have no bad feelings about it at all."

· · · · ·

She tells me now that she had a "pretty normal" childhood "for that time and age," except for being Jehovah's Witness. She was the only Witness in her three-school school district, so when all the other students were coloring pictures of Santa Claus, Lily wasn't. It's not allowed by her religion because it's considered putting a false idol before God.

But sometimes her teachers encouraged her to color anyway, and she did.

". . . Therein comes some of that conflict, you know, where, okay, you've just colored in Santa at school. At night you're laying in your bed thinking," she inhaled deeply, "I wonder if God's gonna be mad at me because I've done this? You know, there's just that whole childhood worrying about whether you're being good or whether you've done something you shouldn't have done, even though it's so innocent as coloring a picture."

Yeah, I know. But I didn't have that problem as a kid. I have it as an adult.

Jehovah's Witnesses also don't celebrate birthdays, so Lily wasn't invited to her friends' parties. "Of course, my friends would say, 'We're really sorry you can't come to this birthday party.' And I'd say, 'Oh, it's not a big deal.' And of course it was, but I just learned how to blow things off. And just let them kind of run past me without feeling—" Lily stops, thinks, and searches for the right words.

Even without the words, I understand. It was no big deal, when

I was a little kid, filling out elementary school forms and writing "deceased" under "father's name," even though the other kids looked at me funny and asked me what deceased meant. If anything, I think I liked that I knew a word that they didn't—like I was smarter or worldlier or something.

"I didn't feel too bad about it. I knew enough to know that it was for my religion, and it was what I was supposed to be doing, so I didn't—I didn't let myself feel sorry for myself."

Yeah, I understand that, too.

"And I have nothing really bad to say about my experience as a Witness, because I learned a lot of good things from it. I learned how to be patient, because when you're waiting for Armageddon to come, you know, there's not a lot you can do except be patient."

And worry.

Lily says she spent her childhood worrying about the "last days" and whether she'd be "good enough" to live through them. Maybe that's because by age thirteen, she was inserting the smooth handles of hairbrushes into her vagina, while fearing she was breaking her hymen and worrying that her future husband wouldn't believe she was a virgin.

But right after telling me that she "learned a lot of good things" from her religion, she tells me that she feels like it's a "cult-type religion, because of the aspect that you can never really have close friends in it."

When she was married to her first husband, and she was "really frustrated" that he never wanted to touch her, another man, who wasn't a Witness, was hitting on her at work. "And I could not go to any of my friends who were Witnesses and say, 'Gosh, you know, I really want to have sex and this guy's like hitting on me, and I'm really thinking about doing it with him,' because they would then immediately feel obligated to go to the body of elders and tell them that I was having these feelings. See? So you couldn't confide in anybody, because you would immediately be turned in.

"And then the body of elders would meet with you and have this conversation with you. . . . So that kind of makes you really not be able to express yourself."

Oh, boy, I really understand that.

"And, plus, Witnesses are not encouraged, in fact, they're completely discouraged from making friends with people who are what they call 'of the world'—people who are not Witnesses, because they use that scripture, you know, bad associations spoil useful habits. And that's just a way of controlling you. It's not good, not good at all."

Oh, yeah, some of my family don't approve that I have atheist friends. It's as though they fear that my friends will convert me away from God. I just tell my family that I'm trying to convert my friends. I'm not sure they buy that. I'm not sure that I do either, but I think my atheist friends do. Rose is an atheist. I think she thinks I'm trying to convert her.

Maybe she's right.

. . . . .

Lily stood in the home she shared with her first husband. "If you can't satisfy me," she screamed, "I'm going to find somebody who will!" She strode out of the house and to the nearest telephone. She dialed the number of one of the men who had been flirting with her at the store. "Come and get me."

He did; they had sex.

Two days later, on the way home from dinner at her parents' house and ravaged with guilt, Lily told her husband she'd slept with another man.

She becomes serious and silent as she relays this to me. She'd expected her husband to be angry. Instead, he looked at her and said, "I forgive you."

Lily stops, as if she's still in disbelief, then lets out a squeak, which seems to express her reaction. "I was just so taken aback. I had no idea what to say. And when we got home we had sex."

"Really?" I calmly remark.

"Yeah. And isn't *that* odd." And she lets loose with a cackling chuckle.

"When you were taken aback, were you, gee, this guy loves me so? Or, gee, *does* this guy love me?"

"No, no. Actually my thought—I think the thoughts running through my head were, oh, no . . ." Her words become chaotic stops, starts, and stutters, until she eventually explains that from the Jehovah's Witness point of view, one is married for eternity, even after Armageddon and all the wicked witches—"everybody but the Witnesses"—are destroyed. At that, Lily chuckles again.

Then she states that she didn't want to live eternally with her husband if they weren't having sex.

"So I think in my head I was thinking, okay, I'm going to have adultery with this man. It's all going to come out, and he's going to divorce me, and then I can find somebody who *does* like sex, okay. But the fact that he forgave me negated that."

So they went home, and they had sex.

Afterward, he turned to her and said, "You know we're going to have to go and talk to the elders about this."

• • • • •

Again, Lily's words begin to pong from one thought to another, as if she's approaching an uncomfortable topic. She eventually gets out that she was a cute, vivacious, popular twenty-year-old, listening at the door to hear what the brothers said to her husband. "And I could hear them telling him things like, 'What is wrong with you? Why aren't you taking care of your wife's needs? Because we talked to her and she told us that she wants to have sex with you and that you're waiting *months* to have sex with her in between times. We just don't get this. Are you masturbating?'"

Her husband promised the brothers he'd do better. And the elders placed Lily on silent probation, meaning she couldn't participate in church meetings until they believed she'd truly repented, but no one but the elders, Lily's husband, and she would know she was on probation. So Lily and her husband went about their lives . . . for six weeks.

Then, desperate because she knew things weren't going to get better, she cheated again with the intention of getting rid of her husband.

"So, of course, when I told him I did it again, he wasn't nearly as forgiving." Her voice is a whisper, but it's a whisper that sounds like it has a bit of a smirk to it. Then she lets loose with that wild cackle. Boldly grinning, she loudly announces, "He was really pissed actually. And the brothers weren't very happy either. They told me I wasn't very repentive and that they were definitely going to have to disfellowship me."

That meant no one from the church could have any contact with Lily—not at church, not at home, not at the grocery store, not anywhere.

Lily knew, though, she could get back into her church. All she had to do was go to three meetings a week, every week, for one year.

"And you have to sit there in the very back. No one can look at you. They can't make eye contact with you. They can't talk to you. They have to completely shun you, but you have to show up at every meeting to show that you *really*," she says the word slowly, "want to do what's right and you really want to be back."

To me, that sounded a lot like the punishment Sadistic Bastard had described when a Master punished his slave for not having his dinner ready.

"It's really difficult to put yourself through it and get dressed and see your best friend's little girl, who was only two at the time, come running to me like this," Lily stretches out her arms, "and then she got *jerked* back. I mean, that—that's a—that's a really difficult, really difficult experience."

I think about how I'd feel if my five-year-old cousin were jerked away from me. I couldn't handle it. I'd break.

"But I did it," Lily says. "And I knew I would do it. *But* I was divorced from my husband, so I was freed from him, which allowed me to hunt for someone different, who I thought would be really good for me." She deliberates for a second. "And so I rushed into a marriage with the Frito chip guy."

Lily ponders for a moment before realizing that she didn't really immediately marry the Frito chip guy. "Actually I dated a bunch of guys and I had sex with every single one of them, for like about four or five months."

"While you were going to church every Sunday?"

"Oh, yes. Yes. Every meeting. *But* I was disfellowshipped. And, you know, for some reason, in some way in my head I thought, *Okay, well, I'm not actually a Witness right now.* And you know what? These guys were asking me out, and I don't think I consciously thought these things, but I've really gone over it over the past thirty years. I've thought about it a lot, and I can see what my actions really meant. In that, I felt, um," she reflects "very," she speaks slowly, "unwomanly or something. It's like when I was dating, I was trying to prove to myself that I was desirable. . . ."

Unwomanly. Desirable. I could feel the words in my soul.

Chapter 25

· · · · ·

I was either in my late teens or very early twenties when a boy I'd had a crush on since high school announced to me that I'd never get a man because I was too strong a woman. I had to stop being so strong, he said. I informed him that I had no intention of not being a strong woman because the stronger I was the stronger a man I'd get. Not surprisingly, he and I never dated.

In my early thirties, a married man I did date—Spinach Man—constantly told me I needed to lose weight. I weighed about 130. Not skinny, but certainly not obese. Maybe that's one of the reasons I never was sure I loved him.

In my late thirties and twenty pounds heavier, I took one of my best friend's children to the beach. My friend's son, who was still in elementary school, looked at me on the hot Galveston sand and simply stated, "Suzy, if you want to get a man, you've got to stop wearing blue jeans and cowboy boots and start wearing short skirts."

I was wearing my bathing suit at the time, so maybe he meant that as a compliment—that I could get away with wearing short skirts. But at that moment, it didn't feel like a compliment. It felt like that boy I'd had a crush on who'd told me I needed to stop being strong. I kept wearing blue jeans and cowboy boots.

I wore them until I started hanging out with a woman who constantly exercised and ate right . . . and who turned men's heads as they begged her for dates . . . and begged me to get her to date them. I started exercising, too, and my weight miraculously plummeted from more than 150 pounds to 118. I was so thin—and couldn't gain weight no matter how many hamburgers, French fries, Hostess cupcakes, and chocolate chip cookies I ate—that friends and family worried I was sick, dying even, and begged me to go to the doctor. Instead, I bought a short dress. I felt like a slut in it. It wasn't me. I went back to Levi's, though I did chuck the cowboy boots for Cole-Haan loafers.

As much as I longed to be womanly and desirable, the things I felt I had to do to be such just didn't suit my soul. Still, I always felt something was missing, just out of reach, like my fingertips were fumbling in the dark, like I wasn't really, truly, fully myself in those shapeless, sexless clothes.

· · · · ·

After the four or five months of sleeping with six or seven men just to make herself feel desirable, Lily married the Frito man. She left him "on the day that he told me if I didn't shut my mouth he was going to kill me, and I really believed that he would." She moved to a West Texas oil town, where she met her third husband. They were married for nineteen years, "although we separated at seventeen years."

Lily then stops to tell me that her mother didn't talk to her about sex or relationships until just before her first wedding night, when she got a "sort of" description about what was going to happen. "Although by that time, I kinda knew what was going to happen because even though I was really naïve, my worldly boyfriends had kind of educated me on some stuff."

Her conversation meanders before she finally admits, "I'd already had oral sex before." Then she smiles and says, "Yeah, actually the first sex I ever had was anal sex."

"Really?" I say casually.

Lily was seventeen, dating her "second major boyfriend," and he *really* wanted to have sex.

"No, no, no, I'm not having sex with you," she protested. "I'm a Witness, and right now, if I got pregnant, that would be like . . . the . . . worst . . . thing to ever happen to me, period."

They kissed. They petted. And he said, "You know, my brother says that he and his girlfriend kind of have sex this way." He explained anal sex.

"Really?" Lily responded. There was curiosity in her voice.

"Well, do you want to try it?"

"Do you think it's going to hurt?"

"Well, how am I going to know that?"

And with me, Lily laughs, a rasping laugh that stretches like chewed gum from her throat to her chest, before it morphs into that joyous cackle. She cracks into a tortilla chip and says we haven't *even* gotten to all of her good stories yet.

I laugh. I definitely want to know more.

When Lily finally had intercourse for the first time, which was on her wedding night, she was nervous, excited, and especially worried. "But when I did bleed, I was really pleasantly surprised," she laughs, and whoops, "Shoo!"

Her wedding night consisted of a little bit of kissing, "and then he stuck it in."

And Lily bites into a chip.

"Of course, the whole time I was married to my first husband, I never had an orgasm. Never."

"I take it you and your husband never did anything like oral sex or anal sex or anything like that?"

"God, no. He wouldn't even let me touch him. . . . He would not let me put my hand on him at all. I never felt of his dick. I never felt of his balls. I never—No, he would not let me do that at all.

The sex we had was very dry sex. I mean, you know, I wasn't even excited. It would hurt a lot of times."

I wince, knowing the pain too well.

· · · · ·

"So when did bisexuality enter the picture?"

"Um, . . . I was working at that Quick Market." She read the store's copies of *Playboy* and *Penthouse* and found herself getting excited over the women's breasts. That, she says, was her first clue, though she thought her excitement was "perverted."

"Of course, I was really into the whole Witness mode then."

Then husband number two brought home some adult magazines that contained photographs of threesomes—all male/female/female, of course. "And I remember thinking, oh, that's really kind of odd. You know, I knew it had happened, but I wasn't really that turned on by seeing it."

After she divorced him, she dated a man who thought a ménage à trois "would be a really fun thing to do." So one night, Lily went to happy hour with a female coworker and whispered her boyfriend's desire. The coworker thought they should go over to his apartment right then, get undressed, and "watch his face."

And that's what they did—as well as climb in his bed and have sex with him. At the boyfriend's request, Lily and her female coworker had sex, too. "But I didn't go away thinking, oh, this is what I'm going to be into."

Later, a different boyfriend encouraged Lily to have sex with a lesbian. "And I felt really uncomfortable. Part of it was her personality. And part of it was since I had no clue what I was doing, it was really kind of confusing to me. And it seemed like it was a whole lot more effort than I really wanted to spend."

She stirs sugar into her tea. "Um, but it didn't turn me off to it. But I didn't know if I would ever, you know, have another experience with a woman."

But when Lily moved to Austin, she had what she called a "little" affair with a woman. "And that was the first time that I found that you could do something like that with a woman and have it be a real turn-on."

Through her, Lily met a twenty-year-old named Emma. Lily, Emma, and Lily's third husband became sex partners. And Emma became Lily's lifelong polyamorous lover.

Lily doesn't need to explain to me that "polyamorous" means loving many. Months earlier, Rose told me she's polyamorous. In Rose's practice of polyamory, it signifies a rejection of monogamy by being sexually active with several partners, but being truthful with each partner regarding her lack of monogamy. What separates polyamory from one-night stands or swinging is having some sort of an emotional involvement with the partners. Rose at the very least cares for each one.

"Like even though I do like women, uh, I'm not one of those people who, you know, sees a woman and, well, I can see a woman and go, oh, honey, look, 'cause I like breasts," Lily says with a grin. "So even though I do like to look at women, normally I think of women as people to relate to as friends, you know. . . . It's not like with men." But Emma was different. "I thought, You are just the cutest thing."

Still, Lily worried. She was a mother who was fourteen years older than Emma and knew there could be repercussions if she made a move that was rebuffed. "I'm very, very aware that you don't ever want to put your children in jeopardy in any kind of way by your inappropriate acts. . . . I mean, your children are your legacy, and you just don't want to mess with that at all."

"But they all know about your lifestyle?" I ask.

In the 1990s, a friend of Lily's dated a man who practiced Dominance and submission. The friend detailed their D/s play for Lily. "And I immediately felt excited, drawn to it." She and Emma began to experiment with spanking, hot wax, and bondage. Then when Lily and her third husband divorced, she started exploring BDSM through the Internet. The following year, she began checking out the local BDSM scene and eventually joined the local BDSM council and became head of its member services.

"Well, they do now," she says.

Her son learned about her lifestyle after her daughter—who is a Domme—left out her own whips and floggers in her bedroom.

"So did you know about her—"

"Of course," Lily chuckles.

While I'm aghast that her daughter is a Dominatrix, her son thought it was funny.

Lily then grows serious. "It's amazing, you know, when you find that your children are sort of having these same things that you do." Both of her daughters are bisexual. She thinks her son is, too, though he says he's gay. "You wonder whether it's genetic. I say it's genetic. It's gotta be because. . ." She pauses.

Lily then tells me that when her daughter was seventeen years old, Lily caught her daughter and a friend binding a teen boy to a chair. At the time, the kids knew nothing about Lily's BDSM life. "Nothing," she repeats for emphasis.

Later that night, in kitchen conversation, Lily's daughter said, "He likes to be tied up, Mother. We were just doing it because he likes that."

Cautiously, Lily chose her words, not wanting to reveal too much. "I understand that people like to be tied up, but you have to be really careful not to hurt somebody and to make sure that you're not doing it against their will, you know."

The girls swore they'd never tie anyone up against their wishes. "In fact, you know, we were thinking it might be kind of fun to be a Dominatrix."

Oh, my God, Lily thought. She said, "Well, you know, I mean, if that's what you're into, I can kind of, you know, I'm not, you know . . ."

Lily breaks into one of her cackles as she repeats this to me.

All I say is a calm "Okay."

"In fact, I have a little flogger that y'all might find interesting," she said to them.

"Did you really?" I say in almost disbelief.

"Yeah, they were almost eighteen."

"Um-huh."

"And they said," Lily's voice nearly hushes with awe, " 'Really?'"

"Yeah," she answered them. "It's sort of—it's sort of—it's sort of a sexual toy."

"Ew!" the girls reacted. "Maybe we don't want to see it."

But Lily's daughter later admitted that she really did want to see the flogger. It was long and rubbery and brightly colored like a Koosh ball. At first, her daughter released another "ew." Then she added an "oooh," and "I want one of those."

Lily told her she wasn't going to give her one until she was of legal age. "There's no way."

"Of course, I'll be using it for different stuff than you use it for, Mother."

"I don't know what they thought I used it for, but obviously she didn't think that we were kinky. She probably thought we were just like playing around, you know."

Lily admits to me that her friends would be appalled to know she gave her daughter a flogger for her eighteenth birthday. "But, you know, I—it wasn't—it's, it's, it's not that big of a deal. It's not like I went out and got her an anal plug or something."

This time I'm the one who cackles and can't stop.

After her daughter received her flogger, she asked Lily what she used hers for.

"Parents are not always as not into stuff as you might think that we are," Lily answered.

The look on her daughter's face conveyed interest. So Lily told her that there were educational groups that were interested in "that sort of stuff" and she could give her some information.

Lily's daughter later joined the local BDSM mentoring program, which, just as it indicates, educates and mentors beginning BDSMers into the Lifestyle.

"I told her if she really wanted to learn stuff that she needed to learn safety . . . because there are so many diseases out there and so many ways you can catch stuff. I tried to explain to her about how, you know, you need to get shots for hepatitis A and B. . . . You don't *have* to do it, but it's a good idea because if you're involved with people, like let's say you have a submissive who really likes to have you put an anal plug up their ass, you know, you're gonna come in contact with some bodily fluids that you normally wouldn't come in contact with, and even though you've got gloves or whatever, you still have to think about the safety issues of that. And so it's better to go ahead and get vaccinated for anything that you might get exposed to. Of course, I tend to be really, really safety conscious, and I don't play—"

And as I think, *Eew, I'd never thought of that*, my recorder runs out of tape. Lily and I have talked that long. So I chuck it and pull my yellow legal pad closer to my chest, grip my black uni-ball pen even tighter, and write that Lily doesn't play with people she doesn't know well. She then begins to tell me about her "boy" luke: luke is actually a grown man, but she calls him her boy because he's her submissive, which is also why his name is spelled in all lowercase.

Every Wednesday, Lily leaves her house and drives over to luke's, where she picks him up for dinner and an evening of running errands, with luke always walking to her left and one step behind her.

Lily then explains that a sub can approach her, but the Domme is the one who courts—yes, courts—the submissive. He can call her "Ma'am," but not "Mistress" unless she has collared him.

And as we talk on, our conversation turns to masks.

Those BDSM masks—black leather hoods often spiked with steel—terrify me. As I say that to Lily, she leans in to me. With excited interest in her voice and a grin on her face, she says, "Why?"

My mouth gapes open. My head shakes. I am speechless. I'm speechless because I don't know the answer to her question, and her teasingly flirtatious grin terrifies me and excites me.

· · · · ·

That excitement is still with me as I climb into my car. But as I push the gearshift into reverse, I realize I have a slight, gnawing headache. I later phone Rose and chat with her about Lily. As we talk, I comprehend how warped my conversation with Lily had been, at least to this Southern Baptist–reared girl—butt plugs, fisting, pride that her daughters are both bi Dommes and that at age thirteen her son dressed as a Dominatrix for Halloween.

Then again, Lily had talked about wrapping someone in Saran wrap. And as she had, all I could think about was Marabel Morgan's *The Total Woman*, a Christian book that came out in 1973 and taught women how to be godly women to their husbands—get naked, wrap oneself in Saran, and greet one's husband at the door. I never dreamed that a BDSM act was being touted as a Christian thing to do to be a godly wife.

It's all so confusing. Since meeting with Lily, I haven't been able to sleep and my headache has only worsened.

And I fear that I could be wrapped in Saran. And I fear that I would let Lily tie me up . . . because, for some reason, I trust her. Her smile had shined like soft moonlight enticing teenaged skinny dippers into warm waters. She was just so damned warm, inviting, bordering on magnetic.

Chapter 26

. . . . .

Maybe I'm too jaded when it comes to romance. My ideal is depicted in the film *Network*, starring Faye Dunaway and William Holden. Dunaway plays Diana Christensen, an unmarried television network producer in New York City. Holden is Max Schumacher, a married network executive. I was living in New York, working for *Fortune* magazine, occasionally lunching at ABC, and dreaming of someday being a producer myself (as well as novelist), when the film came out in 1976.

So it should be no surprise that on a cold November day, I sat enraptured in a Columbus Circle movie theater as I watched Dunaway's and Holden's characters making mad, passionate sex. Maybe I should actually say that she was having mad, passionate sex. He lay there quietly doing his sex job, while she was on top gloriously shouting TV ratings and market shares.

Right then I thought, *If I can find a man who will talk stock quotes with me while having sex, I'll have found my man.*

"IBM went up six! Time, Inc., ten!" And I release a scream of excitement.

Yeah, I know. I have a fantasy after all—a stock market fantasy.

But my point is that Jessica, the young woman who had been fucking numerous random men she'd met on Craigslist, apparently wanted *You've Got Mail*—she'd just written me that she was reading Wynn's emails "a thousand times" and her stomach was flip-flopping over him—and I, the menopausal fifty-year-old who hasn't had sex in almost ten years, want *Network*.

Yep, there you have it—the truth, the confession, the embarrassment. I haven't had sex in nearly a decade.

A "friend" once told me that no man would ever want to date me because of my lack of sexual experience and expertise. At our ages, she said, and we were in our forties, men expect and want women to know what they're doing when they're having sex. I thought, *Well, yeah, but I'm not used, worn-out goods. I don't need all my fingers and toes to count the number of partners I've had and maybe some men find that attractive, because I know I'm not attracted to a man who has stuck himself into every Jane, Mary, and Karen. Hell, I'm not sure I need all my fingers and toes to count the number of times I've had sex.* But what I said was "Yeah, well, this way they can teach me to do exactly what they like and the way they like it done." And I smiled.

She said they don't want to teach, they want to do.

In that case, I'm up shit creek . . . unless I learn something amazing through my research.

· · · · ·

"hang on," Jessica emailed. "i think he's here, meaning i should go, meaning i'll write more later. is it him? . . . yes, more later."

The "more later" included telling me that she and Wynn had sex for hours that night. Jessica visualized her favorite scene from her favorite pornographic story. Her brain went "crazy, flim-flamming around like it's no one's business," until she was able to settle her focus "on that one particular moment in that one particular story," and she orgasmed—"perhaps the most intense orgasm i have EVER had with someone."

Lord. I was beginning to feel like I was reading a romance novel. They cuddled. They stared into each other's eyes. He ran his fingers through her hair. *Yuck.* I turned to Dusty, who continued to detail for me one of his solo enema sessions.

"I took a soap stick deep into me. The pain was intense for a few minutes. It felt so wonderful."

Yes, I understood that Dusty's father had abused him. Yes, I understood that abuse seemed to be a recurring theme in my sex freaks. But I still didn't understand why enemas. Why not floggings? Why not kicks in the groin like Al's friend? Was it because enemas were perhaps the ultimate shame? Certainly, Dusty had expressed that part of him was ashamed of this craving he'd had since he'd taken his first enema fix in his twenties.

But I didn't ask him those questions because too many men told me that they jacked off to my questions and they begged for more. I was tired of men getting off while I was trying to conduct business. So I just thought about Dusty and his French-cut panties and lace bra. Was acting like a woman the most demeaning punishment of all? As though these men deserved the fiery pain and suffering of femaleness? Or were they longing to be feminine because being a woman was so good—or so much easier—in the male mind's eye?

I especially wondered that after hearing again from Robin, my Washington, D.C., cross-dresser.

"If I were asked exactly why I dress, it's probably a reaction to the attention my sister got for being so pretty," she wrote. She repeatedly described her sister, of whom she "may have been very jealous," not only as pretty, but "far beyond" Robin's intellect. Her sister, like their father, had gone into medicine.

In fact, time and again, as our conversations crossed the months, Robin returned to two topics—her lack of confidence, which she described as feeling inadequate, and her father. She constantly professed deep respect for him—and I believed Robin—but she also said he was controlling and passive-aggressive. He never communicated directly with anyone. When he did express himself, he did so in "scorch the earth outbursts." He told Robin's mother, "There are three acceptable responses: Oh Sir, No Sir and Yes your highness."

Robin stressed that her mother, who graduated first in her high school class, "married into a role of high status 'doctor's wife,'" despite not having gone to college. "Not bad for her, coming off welfare as a kid and married into a comfy life."

"Oh Sir. No Sir. Yes your highness." Oh, yeah, that sounds comfy, I facetiously thought.

"Perhaps my mother would have been more supportive of my cross-dressing needs, if my dad were not around. I have corresponded with many CDs, and about ¼ to ⅓ had mothers who bought them whatever they needed in girls clothes," she said.

Yet, when Robin was fifteen and caught cross-dressing, her mother declared, "We do not want a queer son." Robin believed her mother was only speaking the thoughts of Robin's father. "In 1965, no one really knew the difference between a cross dresser and gay. The emotional needs/drives of a CD are very different from a gay. . . . A gay doesn't dress like a girl to attract a guy. A CD dresses to relieve complex stress reduction needs and to explore the way the opposite sex would be."

· · · · ·

Were my Levi's and cowboy boots or Cole-Haan loafers a repression of my sexual desires? Or me just being me: a Texas preppy?

Robin—or rather Rob—was maybe ten years old when he saw a female friend of his parents' dressed in an evening gown that sensuously accentuated her curves. Settling his gaze on her, he felt what he described as a "deep stirring"—the sexual longings of a young boy attracted to a woman.

I think I felt the same thing as a child sitting in the darkness of the Pines movie theater watching Elvis Presley sing "Return to Sender." I remember his unbuttoned black shirt and tight black pants as well as Rob remembers that woman's evening gown and the way it draped over her body. Maybe Elvis is why most of my professional wardrobe is black and I always wear slacks.

· · · · ·

Rob remained a virgin until he met his wife when he was twenty-four years old. Within a month of their meeting, they gave each other their virginity; less than eighteen months later, they married.

"I recall that her grandmother got her a nice nightie with tons of silky fabric. She was uneasy about wearing it and threw it out. I was heartbroken about that. But, we never talked about what she wore. She made it very clear, no gifts of clothing. She had no clue that sexy clothing could enhance our relationship."

Decades later, Rob dreamt about his wife wearing such things. "I'd wake up with a huge erection and needed sex immediately. I'd usually just let it pass. After months of this, I gave her a picture of the corset I wish she'd worn under her wedding gown."

He sent me a picture of the corset. It was creamy and tastefully sexy in an elegantly tailored way. I thought it was beautiful.

But Rob lamented that his wife maintained that she has "no fantasies and no expectations of a sexual nature."

Despite that statement, he later acknowledged that he and his wife frequently have intercourse, though he would like "a lot more passionate times."

"She is orgasmic only orally or manually. She has powerful orgasms and I'd like to be inside her when she's arching her back and coming so powerfully. I have tried to broach the subject, even buying the book 'Mutual Orgasm.' To a certain extent, she's clueless about sex. I have tried to introduce the topic of fantasy, to see if there's something she'd like to work with or from. She continues to say, 'I have no fantasy.'"

IBM, up six!

"It's sort of hard to add to our relationship when she's so disconnected. I'm not a genetic female, but dream about being one from time to time. All I can say is if I were the female and did not have an orgasm during intercourse, and if my husband was asking to work on our relationship to enable that to occur, I cannot think of anything more romantic. But, this is probably not going anywhere. . . . A void in my life."

·　·　·　·　·

"My gosh, she has orgasms!" I wanted to yell at Rob. "Do you know how many women don't? Why are you trying to make her feel less of a woman simply because she can't have the kind of orgasm *you* want her to have? You should be shouting from the rooftops, 'My wife has orgasms! *Powerful* orgasms!'"

Another part of me was sympathetic, thinking what a sweet, kind, loving husband he was that he wanted to help his wife and, unlike so many other men, was willing to communicate with her about their sex life.

But I also wondered if maybe she didn't know how to communicate with him about sex. Maybe she didn't know the words or language. Maybe—since she'd only been with him—she didn't know what she liked or, as Amanda might describe it, what was available on the sex smorgasbord. So she had no way of telling her husband what he wanted to know.

I have no fantasy.

Well, maybe I did have a fantasy other than *Network* sex—an actual romantic fantasy. After hiking the Appalachian Trail the summer after I graduated from high school, I used to dream of a tall, gorgeous, dark-haired man (I never knew who he was or his specific features) helicoptering us to the top of the Smoky Mountains, where we'd spend a sun-drenched day among the wildflowers, picnicking and making love.

Ugh. The mere thought of that makes me cringe. And I hear another movie in my mind—Bette Midler in *The Rose.* In it, she and her lover are watching a movie with an ooey-gooey, mushy scene. At that, she covers her head with blankets and says, "Wake me when the shooting starts." That's the way I feel when I think of my Smoky Mountain fantasy. But it's a fantasy I abandoned long ago, probably about the time I stopped praying for a boyfriend. And I guess I gave up on that prayer about the time I lost my virginity and gained my master's of business administration degree.

Like me, Robin's wife spent the 1980s earning an MBA. Robin then talked her into buying a girdle to wear under her business suits. "She wore it a bit, as did I."

She did more for Robin than I would have.

"It's what I'd wear if I were a bride," she said. "I am, perhaps, very romantic. I'd dress to seal the marriage by making our wedding night so special that he could not forget."

Robin's wife doesn't know about the cross-dressing.

"That must be tough," I said, "keeping such an important part of yourself secret from your most significant loved one for so many decades."

"It is indeed," she replied.

I understood that better than she knew. It was one of the reasons I'd been in therapy off and on for decades. I ached for someone to teach me how to integrate the person who was family-approved with the one I hid from them—the one who drinks, who swears, who longs . . . for touch, for sex.

"The insight into my wife's feelings has led me to keep this a secret," Robin said. "It would be great fun to go out somewhere fancy, both of us in our evening gowns. I don't know if I will ever have that dream come true."

I doubted, too, that my family would ever accept the real me.

But I couldn't allow myself to dwell on me. I had work to do. I printed out Robin's emails and began retyping them into my computer. That helps me to really hear what my interviewee is saying.

As I typed, I was stunned to realize that when Robin was in her forties, she considered undergoing sexual reassignment surgery (SRS)—a sex change.

Around that same time, a friend of hers confessed that he was about to have SRS. Robin's family had been around the friend, knew about the impending surgery, and made clear that they didn't want to have anything to do with the person. Because of that, Robin kept her own desires secret and dismissed any idea of ever having SRS.

As I mulled that over, as well as everything else Robin had emailed me, I read so much sadness. Or maybe it was regret. "Do you see either as a path or theme in your life?"

"Yes," Robin replied, "sadness that I should have tried harder to understand why my academics were not up to par." She returned to her theme of inadequacy. "Maybe if my grandfather had not lost all his money in the depression he would not have become an alcoholic and not have influenced my dad. Perhaps being a girl seemed easier."

And perhaps with that one line—"being a girl seemed easier"—I had my answer.

Robin sent me a link to a women's suit. It was a form-fitting silk suit, the kind my mother wore to church in the 1950s and '60s, the kind Robin wished her wife wore, the kind she imagined wearing as she dreamed of being a woman . . . and as she dreamed of being a bride walking down the church aisle. "It's a great fantasy."

It was also one of the last communications I had with Robin. Over the next few months, we exchanged a few emails, but my emotional connection to her seemed to wither with the summer heat. Perhaps my empathy had been replaced with unrealized irritation that she'd tried to force her wife into becoming Robin's ideal woman, irritation that Robin had been angry and disappointed when her wife had refused. After all, Robin's ideal woman was the perfectly coiffed, pearl-wearing Donna Reed who existed in concept in the 1950s.

If Robin wanted to be a silk-suited, corset-wearing woman, that was fine with me. But the feminist in me rebelled against her wanting to push her wife a half-century backward. Perhaps that's because Robin's displeasure with her successful businesswoman wife ripped too close to the heart of that five-year-old child who wanted to protect her mother. In the 1960s and '70s, I watched too many men try to knock down my mother when she stood straight and strong in their business world. One, I remember, lifted his palm to strike her. She didn't sway, and he pulled back his hand. Others just threatened her verbally.

Yes, being a woman is *so* much easier.

Chapter 27

· · · · ·

"Have you ever been able to actually watch anyone in action or is that something you do not care to do?" Coyote emailed me.

For all my talk of acceptance, and as much as I care for my sex freaks, including Robin, sometimes, I just can't take any more. I need a break from cross-dressing, enemas, slaves, sluts, and whips, and from hearing tales of cheating and from shooing away men I'm not the least bit interested in. I try to disappear from the Internet. I tell everyone I'm not doing any more interviews right now. I say I am writing and transcribing tapes, I'll come back to them with more questions after I finish. And I think I probably really mean that when I'm typing those lines. But in truth, I just need rest. I need distance. I need cleanliness. I need brightness.

Maybe writing about sex isn't so different than writing true crime. Some of the stories I heard had me sitting in my office chair, rocking with anxiety. I couldn't get out of my mind a young woman who'd been raped at sixteen years old. She'd described herself as the daughter of the town tramp who lived on the blue collar side of the highway. Her rapist had been the football hunk with a yachting pedigree. He sauntered away with his crime. She got booted out of her mother's house and had to steal food to survive.

I fretted over another daughter whose mother had been married six times and had had seven kids, many of whom had been taken away by Child Protective Services, most of whom had been adopted out. "There was a man in her bedroom almost every morning, although we never saw them," she said. "We only met the ones she called boyfriends."

Was it any surprise that the daughter had married at age seventeen to get away from her mother, that she'd had three kids, been married three times herself, had insisted on an open marriage in her first marriage, had had numerous live-in relationships, and was bisexual, polyamorous, and into BDSM?

I'm just so tired.

The rape victim stripped her way through undergraduate and graduate schools, earning a master's degree in art. Her work was on exhibit in a prestigious East Coast gallery.

The daughter who'd married to get away from her mother had also earned her college degree, become a physician's assistant, and was finally a happily married mother, though she and her BDSM husband were looking for a poly partner. But their alternative choices seemed to work for them.

Maybe that's why I couldn't seem to do without my sex freaks—sometimes they were inspiring, almost always they were interesting. And as Dusty had said to me after he'd finally finished teasing out the details of his solo enema session, "I guess it goes back to the need to be accepted and understood. . . . I am a normal man in very many ways and all this can be sort of hard to deal with. I am, you see, only human."

And that's what I saw in all of my sex freaks—they were only human. Beautiful, flawed, lonely, hurting children of Jesus, who were fully human, just like me. Sure, they had different issues from me . . . or maybe they didn't. We were all trying to cope and heal from our childhoods, be our wounds scrapes or deep scars. And all any of us wanted was to be loved and accepted for who we are, just the way we are.

So as my friends and family begged me to move on from my sex freaks, fearing I'd be drawn into their darkness—at least what my friends and family saw as darkness—I couldn't. They pulled me. In a matter of days, I found myself clicking on my email and typing, "Hey, Lily Ma'am, how are you doing?" "Amanda, can you explain tantric sex to me again?" "Jessica, where are you? I'm really worried about you."

And within minutes, I typed to Coyote, "Haven't done it so far. Have been invited to. But I had never met the people. So I'm gonna have to wait until I find a couple I trust and I know won't invite me to join, i.e. that they totally understand the ground rules and will stick to them."

I then emailed Rose and told her about Coyote's invitation. "I keep wondering if I should do this. What do you think?"

What was *I* thinking? A true crime writer doesn't need to watch a murder actually happen to write about it. Why did I think I needed to watch sex happening? But it seemed that with each invitation, I was considering it more and more. What was the temptation? Real-life porn? Education? The voyeur in me? To become like them? I didn't understand it. Or could it simply be the professional reporter's insatiable curiosity? For decades, I'd used that excuse with my friends as I'd grilled them about every mundane thought and happening in their lives. They complained that it wasn't a reporter's insatiable curiosity—I was just plain nosey. Could it be as simple as that? That I was tempted to watch others have sex because I'm just a busybody?

Rose didn't think I should watch Coyote have sex—unless I was attracted to him. Otherwise, she said, it would just complicate everything.

I immediately dismissed it from consideration. At least I think I did.

All I know is that my confusion persisted—confusion about so many things, including my role in my sources' lives and my ability to be detached and objective. As much as I desperately yearned to leave myself out of the story, not to expose things about myself that would distress and horrify my family, as well as damage my career as a journalist—after all, there are differing standards of conduct for male and female journalists—the book refused to go in that direction. It seemed to demand more of me, including looking at my own sexuality. I was wanting and not wanting. I was yearning and completely fearing. I think what I feared most was learning—and admitting—what I liked.

By then, Rex had two phone sex sessions lined up and wanted to know if I wanted to eavesdrop again. I declined, citing work. He also had a lunch meeting in the works with a woman he'd met through AFF. ". . . I figure why not? There aren't many things sadder than being married and lonely. And I am lonely."

I was a bit surprised. Not by the lonely comment, but by the lunch meeting. Just a few days before Rex had told me that he didn't know if he was ready to take "the big step" to "physically meet someone."

"Thinking about something like that and actually doing it are two different things," he'd said.

I understood.

"And I couldn't just meet anyone; would have to be friends with them first."

Then Rex started flirting with me.

And I wondered, what happened to men who were turned off by sexually insecure women?

Nine days later . . .

*   *   *   *   *

Rex tugged on a pair of shorts, pulled a black shirt over his head, and laced up his sneakers. He grabbed his keys, climbed into his Firebird, and drove over to the local Saltgrass Steak House.

When he spotted his new "friend" from AFF, he thought she was gorgeous—forty years old, platinum blond hair that hung straight and shoulder-length, brown eyes, and a radiant smile. She wore a white blouse that buttoned down the front and a black skirt. Rex's gaze never made it farther down her body, because it lingered on her full, round figure, just like he liked, and traveled back up to her smile.

As they hugged hello, he noticed the scent of her perfume. It was light and flowery. They sat down at the bar. He ordered a Crown Royal on the rocks. She had a Crown Royal and Diet Coke. They both ordered the prime rib special. She ate more than he did, and she made him laugh. He flirted and made her laugh. She blushed. He thought that was sexy. "You're so pretty," he said.

She blushed again and called him "bad boy."

They stayed later than she meant to, talking about gardening, swimming, her work. She snapped a photo of Rex on her cell phone. They stood in the parking lot and talked more before she moved close to hug him and kiss him on the lips.

He hoped to see her again, soon. In the meantime, he had the sweet scent of her perfume on his shirt. And it drove him crazy.

· · · · ·

While Rex thought about her perfume, I thought about the fact that she'd taken a photograph of him, and I wondered why she'd done that. Again, maybe it's the true crime writer in me, but I wondered if she wanted to use it as a threat to blackmail him. After all, Rex had money. Maybe she'd tell him she'd post it on the Internet if he didn't pay up. Or maybe it was more innocent. Maybe she wanted to show him off to her friends. Maybe she wanted a keepsake memory of a pleasant lunch. Or maybe I had it all wrong and she was just being cautious and protecting herself—she wanted a picture, a record, in case she went missing. After all, before I met Coyote, I emailed a friend his license plate and cell phone numbers in case I went missing.

That night, when Rex's wife got home from work, he handed her the newspaper and made her a drink, just as he always did, despite knowing that whenever she got "even a little drunk," she liked to play the "I have to do everything around here" card.

"Don't get me wrong," Rex wrote me. "My wife has many lovely qualities; otherwise I wouldn't have married her . . . though I am starting to have some doubts about her faithfulness lately. I know, I know, I'm one to talk. But she's not the one who is getting turned down for sex routinely."

Add to that the fact that she spent so much time away from home. . . .

I thought about how Ann Landers, Dear Abby, and just about every other advice columnist I'd ever read had said if you suspect your partner is cheating, he or she probably is. I wondered if Rex's wife suspected he was cheating and if that's why she'd decided to cheat, too. Or if Rex was suspecting his wife was cheating to alleviate his own guilt.

Rex planned on spending the next day running errands with his new girl. He sat with his cell phone waiting for her call. But when it came, she canceled on him. "She started her period today and says that the first day is really bad for her," he typed to me as he chatted with her about how much she liked oral sex and how much he liked performing it. He invited her to come over to his house on Monday, when his wife would be away on a business trip. "I'm going to cook for her and go swimming and whatever else happens. She made no promises and I hold no expectations, but I'm sure she will spend the night and most of the next day here."

My fingers tapped like chirping birds as I typed, "Wow!!! How are you feeling? Excited? Guilty?"

"Excited? Very. Guilty?" he said. "Not enough to make me not want to do this."

"So do a bit of self-analyzing for me," I wrote. I wanted to know what Rex was "saying" to his wife, and to himself, by bringing a potential sex partner into the home and bed he shared with his wife, rather than going to a hotel. To me, that seemed rather passive-aggressive.

Rex said his actions weren't saying anything to her. Instead, they were saying to himself that he was tired of being taking for granted and tired of being sexually frustrated.

So at 3 P.M., he pulled up in front of the home of Courtney, his AFF girlfriend. He didn't go in. "She used to date her roommate, she says, but the way she acts it seems like there is still something going on."

I thought that sounded hinky, but apparently Rex didn't. "I'm certainly not one to talk," he said.

They ran to the bank to make a deposit and to the Big & Tall store to buy a few shirts. As he drove, he caressed her thigh, her arm, her back, her shoulders, anywhere he could touch.

"That feels good," she said. She slipped her hand between her legs to rub herself through her panties.

He eased his hand up her thigh. She pushed it to her crotch and moved her panties aside. He rubbed her private lips and clitoris. "I made her cum before we had to make the next stop." He did it again as they drove to dinner and again as they drove to his house—that time to a "screaming orgasm."

I noted that she'd climaxed in one night more than some women climax in a lifetime. But she was also under the influence of rum—she'd ordered a piña colada along with her steak—and stoned. They'd been smoking a joint as they drove, which was why the last orgasm had been "screaming."

When they finally got to Rex's house, he ensconced her in the master bedroom, dimmed the lights, and made her another piña colada. He handed her her drink and lightly massaged her back.

"Will you take off my skirt?" she said.

He slipped off her black skirt and slowly and gently went down on her. "She was already so wet that it was amazing. I licked her all over, cleaning up all of her wetness."

And I was feeling like I was reading one of his sex stories.

"I ate her for a good long time, about 30 mins. (There was a clock on a table right in my view is how I know.) She says she lost count of her orgasms after eight."

I found it interesting that in the middle of sex he'd watched the clock and she'd taken the time and concentration to count her orgasms. Didn't that distract from the sex?

I guess not. They had intercourse. She came. Rex came. They briefly rested, before he began performing oral sex on her again. "She tastes wonderful"—very mild but with just a little tart—"and is willing to tell me what to do with my tongue to please her, something I love." He ripped open another condom packet and rolled on the rubber.

That time, he didn't come. But as he lay there afterward, she sucked on him.

"It felt wonderful, but it didn't last long. That would be the only complaint that I have of the evening. And believe me, I'm not complaining."

By then, it was late enough that the sun had set and the full moon had risen, so they went for a swim in his pool. Quickly, his trunks came off, her black bathing suit top dropped. She wrapped her legs around him and ground her privates against his until she orgasmed. She then pulled off her swimsuit bottoms and repeated her motions until Rex wanted to sink himself inside her. He resisted. With her hand over her mouth to stifle her scream, she came and plunged herself onto Rex. He couldn't hold back any longer.

"I grabbed her hips and let my lust loose."

Twice more, she climaxed.

"Then I sat her on a step in the pool, took a big breath and went down underwater and started to eat her out. The second time I came up for air, she was screaming into her hand."

Call me jaded. Call me cynical. Call me an uptight, white Baptist girl, but I didn't believe all of this. Oh, I believed that Rex thought all of this happened. I just believed—or at least wondered—if she'd been dramatically faking her excitement. You know, like a contestant on *The Price Is Right* going insanely bonkers just for the opportunity to guess a product's actual retail price and maybe, just maybe, go on to win a prize—like a lawn mower when she lives in an apartment building.

I could see her biting her hand in anguish, just before she thrilled Bob Barker by jumping up and down, bouncing her big boobs until they fell from her tank top, and Bob's foot-long microphone flew upright, and she shouted, "Three hundred, forty-two dollars and seventy-four cents!"

"After catching my breath for only a minute," Rex continued, "she then turned around and put her ass toward me and again started begging me to fuck her. Which I did. She bent down at one point and screamed into the water as I was fucking her like this. I could feel her whole body shudder with that one. And again, through all of this I did not cum."

Maybe he needed me peeking from behind the fence to do that.

They went back inside. He stroked her and kissed her. He went down on her again. And, according to Rex, she came and came.

Briefly, they slept, they had sex again, Rex came, and they slept again until the alarm on his pedometer went off and they panicked that his stepchildren were home. Fifteen minutes later, he drove her the three miles back to her house.

"My pussy is sore," she cooed to him. "But I love the reason it's sore."

"I'm sure you have tons of questions," Rex emailed me.

I always did, but for some reason this time I didn't. Maybe I'd trained Rex so well that he could now anticipate my questions and answer them all without me having to ask him—like an old married couple. Or maybe, I was just worn out from too much sex. He waited almost seven hours before emailing me again. "All those details you like so much, and not a word from you. Guess you are really busy. :)"

And I was. I had other sex sources to deal with.

Chapter 28

•••••

"Good morning, Suzy," Coyote wrote.

"I was just wanting to know if you actually live in Austin. . . . The reason is, sometimes when you meet an individual or couple for the first time, you never really know what you might be getting into. Most are on the up and up and just enjoy plenty of sex. But there are some that are questionable to say the least. . . . You never know when your meeting may be a trap to get you off guard then rob you or worse.

"My whole point is I would like to have a person I could confide in once I have a meeting set up, and let them know as much as I can about who, when, and where the meeting will be. Someone I can trust with this information and know that it will not [be] used for any purpose other than as I have directed. . . . I think YOU are that person, if you are interested. If not, I will understand and it will not hurt our friendship any. I would just feel better knowing that if I should meet with the wrong person or people someday, and something very bad happened, there would be someone who has the answers the police and/or my family will need to know, and hopefully enough information to help catch the ones responsible. Think it over and let me know."

· · · · ·

The strange thing about Coyote and Rex was how my psyche reacted so differently to their cheating. Coyote's cheating didn't bother me. Rex's did. Maybe Coyote's didn't bother me because he was cheating when I met him. And Rex's did bother me because he wasn't physically cheating when we met.

I've had that experience before. When I become good friends with a woman, I usually like and respect her sex partner, as long as they were together when I met her. But if she's single when we get to be good friends and she then starts dating someone seriously, I have a tendency not to like her partner and think he's not good enough for her or, worse, that he's bad for her. Many people interpret that as jealousy—either I'm jealous that my friend is spending time with someone other than me or I'm jealous that my friend is dating someone and I'm not.

I know I wasn't jealous that Rex had slept with another woman. I was disappointed that he'd crossed that boundary into physical adultery. To me, there is a difference between cheating on the phone and cheating in person. Over the phone, Rex wasn't going to infect his wife with a possibly lifelong or life-threatening disease—herpes, syphilis, AIDS come to mind. With in-person sex, he could.

My point is that I don't think Coyote's adulterating ways bothered me as much because he was an adulterer when I met him. Besides, he was a fascinating source, and one of my most beloved sex freaks. So I emailed him that I didn't mind at all being his contact person, I just needed his full name and the name of his hometown.

He sent me his name, hometown, and home phone number with the note, "But don't you dare call this number unless I am DEAD . . . because if I'm not already, I WILL BE . . . Got it???? . . . lol." The ellipses were Coyote's. And I wondered if he'd be forcing me back into writing true crime. If one of my sources died, I knew I'd have to write a book about it, especially if the victim were Coyote.

· · · · ·

Then I heard from Holly, my reluctant virgin.

"To start, I guess I'll introduce you to my mother since most of the things I will be telling you all revolve around her," Holly wrote. "My mother was born to a poor, white trash family where there was a lot of abuse, adultery, alcohol, rape/molestation, and, of course, religious fanaticism. (I only mean that sometimes really ignorant people use religion in the worst way possible—to hurt and humiliate others.)"

I thought about Holly's previous description of her religious upbringing—"very good people," "non-judgmental," "held in the highest regard." Suddenly, that wasn't ringing so true.

"When my mother was a very little girl, her mom told her she hated her and had tried to abort her with a wire hanger. Sometimes I think my mother really hates herself and always has. . . ."

According to Holly, her mother married a wealthy man, whose family wasn't accepting of his bride, and they had three children before the marriage ended in divorce. Holly's mother then married a man named Ed.

"She was in the doctor's office with Ed, waiting to get him snipped so as to never have kids. . . . As she was reading a magazine, she felt in the pit of her stomach a voice asking to be born. Of course this was me from Heaven pleading with her (again, the religion when it fits . . .) to allow me life. SO, she grabbed the dull Ed, and left the office."

Three months later, Holly was conceived. Five years later, two "significant experiences" happened in her life: "1) Ed divorced my mom and left us for another woman. 2) I experienced my first miracle."

I rushed over the miracle mention to note that Holly had written "left *us*," not simply that he left her mother, as if Holly still feels the hurt. Then again, Holly described herself as "a huge Daddy's girl" at the time of the divorce.

To help her cope with her sadness, Holly's mother took her to the pet store, where they picked out a parakeet for her fifth birthday. One day, Holly carried the bird and cage outside and opened the cage door. The bird flew out. Holly screamed. Her mother came running. "When my mom asked what was wrong, I blubbered, 'First my daddy leaves and now my bird.'"

·　·　·　·　·

"I will always be thankful for my mother during these points in my life where I experienced extreme distress," Holly said. "She was always the one to pick up the pieces and tell me it was okay. . . . She walked and walked with me around the neighborhood asking people if they had seen my bird, which of course they hadn't.

"Now the miracle part." About a week later, Holly was playing outside at her elementary school. "It was during recess, and there were kids running and screaming everywhere."

"Come see!" a little girl begged.

Holly did. And there, to her "utter disbelief," was her parakeet. "My little bird had found me. . . . I think God must have known I really needed to see that not everything in life abandons us forever, sometimes they just need to see the world before they come back home." I wondered if I'd experienced a "miracle" like Holly's, if I'd feel differently about men always leaving.

"My sister recalls having this conversation with my mother one day where my mom told her that she would have a daughter who would tell her EVERYTHING and be sooo close to her," Holly continued. "And in fact, my mom did have a daughter who would tell her everything—me."

. . . . .

Like me, Holly had tried to be the daughter her mother wanted. "I listened to her rant about men, read my bible, told her my secrets, gave her advice, held her hand in public, loved her unconditionally as she did me. She was my all."

Holly even returned to her mother after college.

"I had zero dollars in my bank account, had just graduated from art school where I had changed not too dramatically considering, but had learned about pot brownies, how cigarettes made me feel sophisticated, that mixing drinks is a bad idea, that I thought Leonardo Da Vinci was overrated, and that SEX was an all caps word for me. I had never had sex . . . but . . . I thought about it all the time, what I wanted it to be like, and tried to reason internally what I thought sex should be and mean to me. Obviously I am still confused, but I did find some enlightenment. I learned that sex is not wrong or dirty, that it is beautiful in all forms no matter what or who takes part, and that perhaps someday I might like to try it. My mom told me a few days after I returned that she regrets me not having had it at this point—after all—she wanted me to experience everything life had to offer, this is somewhat ironic."

I found it ironic, too, that my mother constantly told me never to do what she had done—live her life for her mother.

"Anyhow, after I returned home, I didn't want to follow her obligingly. I had learned too much that caused me to pause in our relationship. So I decided to leave and move." Holly decided to go east.

Her mother flew across the country to help her move. "She was angry the entire time and threatened to go home midweek. . . . She saw me smoke, and I think she got scared that I was changing already before her very eyes. . . . I began to realize that my relationship with my mother was never going to be quite the same. Three thousand miles was not going to make us closer; it was going to make me detach and see my mother for who she was—not a bad person or someone to despise, but someone whom I needed space from. . . . Without the shadow of my mother, I could then focus my attention on understanding myself rather than seeking validation through my mother."

After Holly's move, the fights with her mother continued, especially as Holly planned a trip home to see her mother *and* her friends. "After all, I should not see anyone else during my trip home." So rather than upset her mother, Holly told her she loved her and canceled her trip. "In not coming home, I had hoped she would realize I wanted to see her more than anyone. . . ." Instead, Holly never heard from her again.

Holly's mother later wrote an email to one of Holly's siblings saying Holly was much more like her biological father, the man who had left them both, than the father who had reared her.

"So this concludes my story for now. I think I've exhausted myself thinking about it. However, this has been very therapeutic since I have ignored my feelings about my mother since our fallout. I know we will speak again. It's just that I am not willing or ready to at this point. Speaking to her means I will have to accept her and not expect anything more out of her than she is capable of giving. . . . She cannot change who she is—she is not strong enough. This was a hard thing for me to accept, that my mother is strong, but not strong enough. It has taught me though to aspire beyond what my mother cannot achieve."

Strong, but not strong enough.

I was living in New York City when I was Holly's age. It hadn't been difficult for me to leave my mother. Like Holly, I planned to achieve beyond my mother, though she achieved immensely. Unlike Holly, my mother had accepted my move. In my family, work has always been an acceptable excuse. I could go anywhere professionally. I could achieve anything professionally. But growing up, separating emotionally, that was unacceptable.

She cannot change who she is.

"Now I have to keep encouraging myself to take the road less traveled," Holly said, "meaning to follow through on the things that scare me the most, but will be my most self-defining moments."

I sat at my computer and thought about that. Sex, relationships— they're what scare me most.

No. What scares me most is mother, family, and men.

Judging me. Leaving me. Hurting me. Rejecting me.

Chapter 29

· · · · ·

"i cannot get enough of this boy," Jessica wrote. "it is so fucking crazy. every time i see him it bowls me over, just sort of floors me. i can't even wrap my brain around it. i hadn't seen him in two days and as we were standing outside, waiting to go to this concert, he said, 'when did two days become so long?' i know. it's insane in the best possible way."

After the concert, they drove to the university where Wynn was a graduate student. In his office, on his desk, they went down on each other. "hot," she said.

"what was hotter though, and is still blowing my mind is the following: wynn was sitting in the chair and i was straddling him. we would kiss, then pull back and look at each other from a distance of about four inches apart, kiss again, pull back, look at each other. we kept doing this and every look became more and more intense that i seriously started to have orgasmic paralysis from simply looking at him. i mean, we had our shirts off but it was just looking at him. i don't even know how long we did this but at one point he whispered, 'my god . . .' and that just set me over the edge.

"this shit is off the hook. . . . i can't even handle it."

I was having trouble handling it, too—my "jealousy" issues. Just a few days before, I'd written her, "Girl, where are you? I feel lost when I don't hear from you. :)."

She'd written back gushing about Wynn. "part of me wonders when i'm going to wake up or how long this can last in its bubble but the truth is that there is so little going on outside of wynn that who knows, it could last forever." She closed with "i just can't believe he came from craigslist. . . . it seems so surreal and so nice and so easy and so fantastically brilliant."

And I was back to Bette Midler in *The Rose*—"Wake me when the shooting starts."

I turned my attention to Coyote. I knew he wasn't going to "betray" me with any serious relationships.

· · · · ·

"I have been looking for a common denominator in all the things related to this lifestyle," he wrote. "I think it is just the RISK involved. I believe in a 'safety net' so to speak, but the risks are definitely exciting."

Ah, risk—it seemed to be a common denominator for so many of us—Jessica hooking up with Craigslist strangers, me going to therapy to try to learn how to do a relationship. But I knew I could more easily adapt to having sex on an office desk than I could to the risk of having a relationship. Faux relationships with my sources did me just fine.

By the next day, Coyote added great sex and variety to his list of common denominators. They, along with risk, were what kept him wanting more. "It's as addictive as alcohol or gambling."

"Do you consider yourself a sex addict? Or a risk addict?" I replied.

"Sex addict," he answered, since most of the risks he took involved sex.

A few days later, Coyote emailed me that he'd received a letter from the Veterans' Administration notifying him that he'd be receiving 100 percent disability due to PTSD. "YeeeeHaaaaaaw," he wrote. He could retire. Then he'd have even more time for sex.

I moved on to Rex.

Rex emailed me that while his wife had been waiting at home for a can of paint for their bathroom, which Rex supposedly was shaking at Home Depot, he'd been meeting Courtney in a bank parking lot. He thought she was falling for him.

"When I think about you," she whispered, "what I'm thinking of is your mouth, your lips, and your tongue on my pussy, eating me out."

Wake me when the shooting starts! I thought. Rex joyously thought he was a sex object to her. And that made him laugh.

But Rex wasn't limiting himself to Courtney. He'd met a married, forty-seven-year-old woman on AFF. He knew she liked to be handcuffed, so he'd written her one of his stories in which he'd 'cuffed her and had his way with her. Soon, he was circling the parking lot of his local Marriott hotel, looking for her.

She dipped her hand inside his black shorts and stroked him. "I want to suck on you," she said. She bent down to him.

· · · · ·

That night, I found myself emailing Rose: "I'm so sick of hearing about everyone else's sex lives but not having one of my own.

"I need to find one of those surrogate sex people who is drop-dead gorgeous and hire him/her to teach me how to be a great lover.

"It's such a dilemma: I don't think I could get involved with anyone who could be a serious relationship but I don't think I could sleep with anyone who I wasn't physically attracted to and who I really, really like."

As I've said, there's only so much risk I'm willing to take in my personal life. And I guess Rose knew that because she didn't respond. Then again, she was in the midst of a serious, heterosexual, monogamous relationship. I was so disappointed. She was supposed to be my one friend who understood and supported my research. Now she was just like all my other uptight, white, vanilla friends.

Was I jealous, too? Probably. I don't mean I was jealous that she had a relationship and I didn't, but I was jealous that she wasn't available to spend more platonic time with me . . . as well as that my formerly bisexual, polyamorous friend wasn't available to me sexually. I guess now's past time to admit what I really don't want to. Oh, God, I really don't want to because of my family.

When I first started researching this book, I asked Rose to kiss me. Never in my life had I been kissed so luxuriously. I wanted to learn how to kiss like that. And I wanted to sample more of that. But with her hetero, monogamous relationship, I knew that would never happen. Let me clarify. I don't mean that I fantasized that Rose and I would have a serious love relationship beyond friendship. I didn't. But I sure did like kissing someone I cared about. To me, that was risk.

Chapter 30

· · · · ·

"The first time I had anal sex was unsuccessful."

That was the heading on an attachment Holly emailed me. In the attachment, she finished the thought: "It had hurt too much to continue."

I had to laugh. In a previous email, she'd provided a dissertation about attempting anal sex with her last boyfriend. And the more I'd read of that email, the more I'd realized that the reason she'd maintained her virginity was because of her very first boyfriend, the one to whom she wished she'd given herself.

"I thought sex would be the ultimate act of love between us and would forever unite us," she'd written about him. "I would then be free to have sex with whomsoever I choose afterwards because we would always belong to one another no matter the course of events following. In my head I know this to be off track, but I can't shake this thought that I missed my chance."

Wake me when the shooting starts.

"I wonder what he would say if he found out I wasn't a virgin if we ever got back together and I had had sex. How terrible is that though—that sex should be a breaking point in a love between two

people. And is it a testimony of my lack of willpower that I want
to just have sex for the sake of experiencing it?"

No.

"Now when I have sex it will be too much a part of my head
instead of my gut where it belongs. I don't want sex to be in my
head. I want to feel it in my heart, my gut, and my crotch. It doesn't
belong in the folds of my brain where enough unnecessary matter
is housed. But there it lies. It is becoming much more than it should
ever have been. It is almost a battle of willpower to see how long I
can maintain this 'virtue.'"

I understood too well about sex being in the head and not the
heart, gut, and crotch. I understood too well the battle of willpower
to see how long I could maintain "this 'virtue.'" But I also knew I
did have to keep sex in the folds of my brain because I had a book
to write. So as I stared at Holly's new attachment, I clicked into
reporter gear and read.

Holly wrote that she eventually succeeded in having anal sex,
and she stressed that her level of sexual experience had increased
with each boyfriend, always on her terms, and always without doubt
or second-guessing. "The moment[s] before any 'new' sexual encounters were always heightened by my own desire and anticipatory
expectation of what was to come. This brings me to my next lead
Suzy . . ."

Holly was the one who typed the ellipses, and they were well
deserved because those three little dots symbolized what I imagined
to be her next three moves. She took a pausing little gasp, then a
long deep breath, followed by a stretching exhale, all preparing
both of us for what she was about to say . . .

"I feel that since talking with you, I have been able to better
understand my own perceptions of sex and what I am willing to
accept about myself. I have always enjoyed sex regardless of the lack
of penetration. This last week I was in NY working, and I got a
chance to do a lot of playing as well. My sister and brother-in-law
have a friend living in NY whom I was introduced to only 2 weeks

ago. He offered to be my tour guide for the week. Whilst guiding me through the city showing me sights such as the teeming streets of Chinatown, the long stroll along the Brooklyn Bridge during the evening, and the restaurants any gourmand would enjoy, he also carried me through my first time having sex, actual penetration."

My eyes stopped moving across the computer screen. Blankly, I stared at her words. Consciously, I had to goad myself to start reading again.

"Suzy, I know this may come as a shock to you . . ."

That was an understatement.

". . . but this past week in NY, I felt very comfortable with taking that next step, albeit with a practical stranger. I liken it to my first time kissing a boy. That was at summer camp when I was 16 and it was the most romantic first kiss. We had snuck out to go sit by the waterfront and he told me Greek mythological stories and as the tide rose up to tickle our feet . . ."

Oh, this was getting too melodramatic for me.

"We moved our position to the nearby docks. I remember him reaching over and kissing me on the mouth, open and with his tongue. It was all I could do to not scream out loud how excited I was to have finally been kissed."

Oh, this definitely was too romance novelish, over the top for me. I can't even remember my first kiss.

"This experience was similar. I never again saw that boy from summer camp, and I don't really care if I ever see this man again, although I hope to because I really did like him, but regardless, I cherish the experience more. I am not in love with this man, I am in love with what he did to me. In my favorite city in the world, in a big white fluffy bed, in a beautiful apartment uptown, with a gorgeous Irishman with long brown hair, I lost my virginity. I had to remind myself to drink in my surroundings."

Drink in her surroundings? When I lost my virginity, I was in utter shock. And all that went through my head was Peggy Lee singing, "If that's all there is, my friend," then there was a big pause in my mind until I continued, "then let's keep dancing . . ."

"The apartment actually belonged to his friend who loved to fish so the place was dressed with fishing paraphernalia. There were lures all around, pictures of him catching huge beasts, and I remember he must have liked maps since he had several adorning his walls."

We were on my little twin bed—no need for a big bed since I was planning on being a virgin all my life—crammed against the wall. A TV my sister and mother had given me was at our feet. It sat on top of a wicker table I had inherited from my Jewish–Christian Scientist grandmother who would have been appalled at what I was doing, just as my mother would have. Next to my right ear, on a wicker trunk that I'd bought at Pier 1 when I was at Baylor, was my answering machine from Radio Shack and a loudly ticking Bulova alarm clock that I'd received for high school graduation. I don't know this because I was in a romantic, take-it-all-in trance. I know it because that clock had metronomed me to sleep for a decade and I'd lived in that apartment with the off-white walls and no air-conditioning for three years.

But Holly had noticed everything, including the two *Breakfast at Tiffany's* posters hanging on the walls—it was her favorite New York film and the first film she saw that made her "adore" New York City.

"You see, I love to fish and I also associate fishing with my father who passed away since that was what we did together during our time alone."

Oh, sheesh. I don't remember any alone time with my father. I remember him standing outside the First Baptist Church of Lufkin, Texas, smoking cigarettes with the other deacons. I stood with my mother, quietly watching him, silently waiting for him, as though he was part of a circle that we women weren't allowed to join. I didn't like that. I remember his Kent cigarettes on the wooden lamp

stand in our den as he watched boxing on a snowy TV. I hate boxing. I remember him eating oatmeal in the mornings before driving
off to work in his green or white (depending on the year) Temple
Associates company car. I hate oatmeal. And I remember how he
used to make so much noise in the bathroom every morning that
he'd wake me. And I remember the morning we were on vacation
in Cripple Creek, Colorado—though I usually have trouble remembering the town's name—when I was *really* angry at him for making so much noise that I couldn't sleep and I *really* wanted to sleep
and, then, KABOOM! I bolted upright in bed, furious at him, not
understanding that the KABOOM! was his dead body hitting the
floor, curled like a child at the foot of the toilet. He was dressed
only in his white boxers. I remember my mother shielding my eyes
as I walked past the bathroom to exit the premises, me not wanting
to look at his dead body, but wanting to look. I glimpsed. That's
how I know exactly where he lay and how he was dressed.

· · · · ·

"Everything felt right. I was completely ready, however a bit nervous. I waited patiently while he went upstairs to get 'something.'
When he returned, he laid me on the bed gently, and told me to
relax. I noticed how the pictures within view were poorly hung;
they were a triptych of colorful pastels with black, slender, lyrical
figures in the foreground. He slowly entered me and he continued
to reassure me. I had asked that we use a towel since I wasn't sure of
whether or not I would bleed (which I did not thankfully). He was
both sensual, erotic, and sweet. I couldn't have asked for a more perfect first time having sex. For the rest of my stay we made love
several more times and each time I felt more aroused and excited
to be doing what I had waited so long to do. He knew I was a virgin
and offered to do anything I wanted since I had 'waited 23 years to
have sex.' It was a fairly capricious decision on my part to have sex
at that moment, but I felt sure of myself and comfortable with my
choice. I have always been sexual even as a little girl. The first time

I had an orgasm was when I was nine. This was one of those rare, self-defining moments and I came out of it with a better appreciation of what sort of woman I've become. I am proud of myself for waiting as long as I did, and for not exploiting my first time with obnoxious and overly dramatized fantasies of love being the deciding factor in having sex."

• • • • •

For me, love certainly wasn't the determining factor. Like Holly, it was more like I just decided to do it, get it over with, get it out of the way. Why? When had my beliefs gone by the wayside? I wish I had an answer for that. I don't.

As I sit here and ponder that—where and when my staunch black-and-white beliefs turned murky gray—I wonder if it was teen-aged rebellion ten years too late. But I don't know that for sure. I do know that that wasn't in my conscious mind. I was twenty-seven years old and in grad school at the time, getting my master's in business administration. And what was in my mind, and what I cried out over and over that night I lost my virginity was "It hurts. It hurts." And I did bleed.

Chapter 31

. . . . .

Twenty-four years later, everyone's life seemed to be changing but mine. And I was having a hard time adjusting to their changes—Holly losing her virginity, Rex cheating. But perhaps most of all, I was having trouble adjusting to monogamy. Rose's. Jessica's. Even Amanda, my very first source, had met a man on AFF and decided she was finished sampling the sex smorgasbord. There were no better "dishes or flavors" than that on which she was already dining, she said.

I'd been researching sex for a full eight months. I'd communicated with hundreds of people. And I was beginning to wonder if kinky, alternative sex *wasn't* AFF or Craigslist or threesomes or cross-dressing. Maybe *truly* alternative sex was not needing a relationship. In that case, *I* was the kinky one. No wonder my shrink and my shrink friend wanted me to have a relationship—they wanted me to be plain vanilla. And the one thing my mother had always taught me was that you don't want to be like everyone else.

Then, Coyote hit me up, again. Good ole dependable Coyote. On the pretense of getting together to educate me about PTSD, he wanted to make sure that I didn't forget that he wanted to "put on a private masturbation 'demo'" for me. "It would mean a lot to me as far as me trusting you and being comfortable with everything I tell you. I don't know for sure why. It just would."

Less than fifteen minutes later, I found myself sitting by myself drinking straight gin. Maybe that was the one change in my life, because that's not something I normally do.

"Man, I need someone to talk to about this book," I emailed Rose. "This is a lot to handle. Folks are emailing me, 'after I talked to you' blah, blah, blah, and it's like some major change in their lives." I felt horrible that Holly had lost her virginity because of talking to me. Helping an unmarried woman work her way through deciding to have premarital sex is not what good Baylor girls—what good Christian girls—do. But I also wondered if sources like Coyote and Rex did things just for me—to entertain, impress, or shock me, or simply to get my attention. "I'm concerned about the effect I'm having on people."

And I was concerned about the effect all of this was having on me. When a friend referred to my sex freaks as gross, I got angry at her, while I feared that if I ever did have the opportunity to have sex with someone I liked, it would take "something major" to turn me on. She thought not. She thought I'd want hot, loving sex.

I disagreed.

Rose emailed me, "For heaven's sake don't let that guy masturbate in front of you!"

I waited until the next day to answer Coyote. "I don't know about the masturbation thing. It might be crossing the line of getting involved with my subject matter, and I just can't do that. I'll contemplate it over the next couple of weeks. But I definitely want to get together again."

In truth, I'm not sure I was considering Coyote's offer. If I were honest with myself, I would have considered it if he were a gorgeous, young hunk of a man. But I wasn't all that interested in watching a beer-bellied retiree with rosacea rub his penis until sperm oozed. Maybe that makes me superficial. It probably does. But, it was also a safe bet, meaning not watching would keep me safe. Though I trusted Coyote . . . well, I'd trusted other men in my life, too, and that hadn't turned out to be a lot of fun.

· · · · ·

I wrote Rose, "Am I a hypocritical Christian?"

I'd recently lunched with a tall, muscularly taut, married, male friend of mine. We'd met at a book event only a few months before. That day, I'd glanced at his brown cowboy boots and stared at his long, blue jean–covered legs, then at his discreet Western belt buckle, followed by a study of his professorial sport coat. Underneath it, he wore a black, chest-hugging, rock-and-roll T-shirt for an Austin band. The palest of soul patches peeked beneath his bottom lip. That gunpowder thumbprint of hair was more Wyatt Earp than rock and roll, though it reminded me a bit of real jazz. I liked the discordant chords of his look.

He said we'd met before.

I didn't remember.

He told me it was at a blues club, at a party for a movie premiere during a film festival. I remembered that. I remembered meeting the friend he said he was with. But I still didn't remember this rock-and-roll, jazz cowboy with the long legs.

He asked me to join him for a drink. We went to one of my favorite restaurants. It had dim lighting and jazz piano that played perfectly with cold Bombay Sapphire martinis, straight up, with a twist. Halfway through my drink, as we talked about my book and sex, I wanted to take him down a back alley and kiss him. Hard. Gin does that to me. But I knew I shouldn't—he was married. We hugged good-bye. I felt like I fit into his body just like a woman should, like I was finally home. I'd never felt that way before.

I avoided him for months, though we occasionally flirted through email. But once the temperature climbed from sport coat and T-shirt weather to T-shirt only, the cowboy and I sat together once again. He made me think of all of my married, cheating, "good" men. I think I was the one who made sure we met this time in a restaurant lighted as brightly as the August sun. I curled my fingers around a cold glass of a Diet Coke.

"Wouldn't it be nice to have a friend to sleep with?" the cowboy said.

I filled my mouth with a bite of spinach quiche. I chewed. I wouldn't let myself look at his long arms, lean with muscles. I thought about how much I love the quiche at this restaurant. I glanced at the women-who-do-lunch and the businesspeople who sat around us. I swallowed. "Yes," I answered and reached for my Diet Coke.

The cowboy's question had come amid talk about how he and his wife didn't have a sex life, that she wasn't interested in having one, blah . . . blah . . . blah. But I'd leaned in and listened closely to his blah, blah, blahs because with him, since I was somewhat interested in him—sobriety had lessened my desire—his clichéd words seemed fresh and new. I wanted to believe them. I wanted to believe *him*.

But I set down my glass of Diet Coke and pulled back. "I have qualms about having premarital sex," I said. Raw in my mind was Rose's response to my question: "Am I a hypocritical Christian?"

I'd hoped, perhaps had even expected, that my simple five-word sentence would elicit a simple, one-word answer: no. And that no from my beloved, trusted friend would alleviate any guilt I had, as if she were a priest who could absolve me of my sin.

"Suzy, what do you care what I think? I'm an atheist!" Rose had written back.

I should have heard in my head my shrink lecturing me that I had set myself up. Actually, I should have heard that before I'd hit "send." But I hadn't.

Though Rose and I had been friends for at least seven years, she said she wasn't "clear on what particular brand of Christianity" I was into. Therefore, she couldn't "accurately" answer my question. She knew the Bible well, she said, and I knew that she truly did. In her youth, Rose had considered herself a devoted Christian. Based on what she knew about the Bible, she said she didn't know any Christians who lived a godly life.

She proceeded to list "the principles that made Jesus famous" but that no Christian she knew lived up to: giving their money and worldly possessions to the poor, turning the other cheek, trying to remove the plank from their own eyes before removing the splinter from others, and, of course, abstaining from sex outside of marriage. "If I knew someone like that," she wrote, "I'd be a lot more impressed with Christianity. If I saw millions of people behaving like that, I might wonder if there's something to it."

I felt like shit. And to answer her question, I cared what she thought because she was my friend, whom I love very, very much, and exactly because she is an atheist. I did—do—want to be a good representative of Jesus. "Gotta clean up my act, obviously," I wrote her.

A week after my lunch with the married cowboy, I hadn't heard from him. I emailed Rose. "I guess he realized he wasn't going to get laid by me and dropped me. I can't believe how this is upsetting me. I guess it was nice to be wanted."

I explained to Rose that our email conversation about Christianity and hypocrisy and premarital sex had been a factor in my behavior. "Ironic, isn't it, that I'm worried about premarital sex when I haven't had any in nearly ten years."

Strangely enough, whenever I think about sex and me and how long it's been since I've had it, all that comes into my head is a TV commercial for Wolf Brand Chili:

"How long has it been since you've had a big, thick, steaming bowl of Wolf Brand Chili?

"Well, that's too long!"

Chapter 32

. . . . .

The Wolf Brand Chili ad played in my head like a bad song. "Well, that's too long. Well, that's too long." Say it enough times and it sounds like a stuck record. "Well, that's too long. Well, that's too long."

I felt stuck. Stuck in my celibacy. Stuck in my faith. Stuck in my family. Stuck in my attraction to married men. Stuck in my fear of men. Stuck in my fear of touch.

Despite the fact that I'd "joked" to Rose about finding a sex surrogate, I was too chicken to go to one. At some time or other, my memory is blurry on the date, my shrink suggested I go to a sex therapist, which I realize is not necessarily the same as a sex surrogate. Still, I wasn't about to go to the woman my shrink had recommended. I'd seen that therapist around town and had observed her being rude to strangers, as if she believed she was better than them. I didn't like that, which made me not like her. It never occurred to me to find another sex therapist, because I knew my family would freak over the idea—and I knew I'd tell them. Don't ask me why. I don't know why. I just knew I would.

Yet I needed something more in my life. Not just my personal life, but my sex research life, too. I wasn't aware of it at the time, but it was almost as if my current sex sources and I were becoming bored with each other and were distancing from each other. I never heard from Holly after she lost her virginity, despite the fact that I'd told her I wanted to stay in touch. I was barely hearing from Jessica. She was so focused on Wynn that she didn't have the time or desire to write. Rex was in a depression over his wife, his marriage, and the fact that Courtney was blowing him off, rather than blowing him—though he had yet to realize that's what she was doing. Dusty said his search for compatible playmates was sucking "so to speak," therefore he had nothing more to add to the book.

The only one who seemed to be staying in touch was Coyote. He *had* used me as his "safe" contact for a questionable sex rendezvous at a motel known for drug dealing. But I went into such a panic when I didn't hear from him until the following day that he never used me again, though he did keep me up-to-date on his sexual activities, *after* they had occurred.

And as fond of Coyote as I was, as I said, I needed something new, something more, something "major" to turn me on. So I sat at my computer, staring once again at Craigslist. Unlike nine months before, I wasn't anxiously, timidly waiting for someone to answer my ad. I was purposely and determinedly cruising. Not for me. For the book. Specifically, I was cruising for swingers. Again, not for me. For the book. I was growing antsy that, research-wise, I hadn't yet dived into the swinging waters.

Yes, I'd interviewed Frank, the swing club owner. But he hadn't been actively swinging since before his wife's death, and I'd been too chicken to go to his club. I'd spent time with Angela and Kai, my BDSM-ing swingers, but since then they'd forsaken swinging for BDSM. Plus, I'd been too chicken to go to their favorite swing club with them when I'd had the chance. There seemed to be a theme here. If I wanted something new, something more, I had to stop being so chicken. "Do it!" I yelled at myself.

I scrolled down casual encounters in San Diego, California.

I spotted the headline AVERAGE MID-LIFE SWINGERS. I stopped. "somewhat fit fun seekers iso [in search of] our al and peg [bundy] type counterparts. we like to eat out, drink up, do some fun average stuff, then come home and mess around." Like Jessica, they didn't write with capital letters. "if you're married and looking for some extracurricular activities maybe we're it."

They also wanted a d/d (drug and disease) free couple who were committed to each other and had a list of swinger rules that they "generally" respected.

I obviously didn't fulfill a single one of their requirements—other than being drug and disease free—but I answered their ad anyway and asked if they'd talk to me about their sex lives. In less than two and a half hours, I received a reply.

"sounds like out of the closet, into the frying pan to us. isn't cl a little lowbrow? why don't you try lifestylelounge.com? now there you'll find the beautiful people by the bushel."

"I'm looking for real people," I responded. "If you consider CL lowbrow, why are you on it?"

"the lowbrow people rock. god damn we've had fun with cl people. but the beautiful people, they cluster together. you can get a bunch of 'em with one net. although we haven't tried. and it's fun to weed through people on cl. that's why we're here."

They soon wrote me again. "what are you wearing? lol."

"Oooh, baby, baby," I typed, while—yes—laughing. "I'm wearing a too-tight polo shirt that binds my breasts and an old pair of Levi's that are unbuttoned several buttons because I've gotten so fuckin' fat! Real turn-on, huh? LOL."

I didn't give a hoot what my shrink thought about my "oooh, baby, baby" research tactics, though she was hassling me right then about my work—telling me my life was out of balance, that I didn't play enough, that I didn't have a good enough support system. But at that moment, talking to who I thought was Amy, the wife, because the email came from her address, and feeling safe because it was the wife and not the husband, I felt like I *was* playing. Finally,

I wasn't hearing—and I wasn't bored by—"my wife won't have sex with me." In fact, on days like this, I didn't want to escape my sex freaks—they made me laugh.

Amy was a forty-five-year-old executive with a nonprofit organization. Her husband, Jack, was a fifty-one-year-old sales rep who loved to build things in his spare time. Born and bred Southern Californians, they'd been married for twenty-seven years and swinging for the past four. "We got started by accident actually," she wrote. And later—much later—I realized Amy sometimes used capitalization, which meant Jack may have been the one who typed, "what are you wearing?"

Uh-oh.

The accident occurred when they invited six of their neighbors over for a barbecue. Amy mixed up a batch of fuzzy navel cocktails, and before she and Jack knew it, everyone was naked in the hot tub. A group grope and much laughter ensued, though one wife got angry and never returned. The others did, and the next time it was "more intense, but no screwing yet." Amy and Jack thus began a soft swing affair with one of the couples and a hard swing affair with the other. "We have a happy marriage and found out in the hot tub that night that mixing new people in sometimes really adds a lot of spice to our sex life. we have sex a lot more than we used to. If your marriage is strong and you trust each other it is fun as hell."

But Amy got sick of their hard swing male companion because he drank too much and wasn't good at foreplay, so she and Jack went searching on Craigslist, which is where they found Nikki and Clay.

· · · · ·

Amy and Jack didn't really expect Nikki and Clay to show up for their "date." They thought the Craigslist couple was just messing with their heads. Nevertheless, they bought new clothes, Jack got a haircut, and Amy got her hair and nails done. They purchased condoms, though they'd never used protection before, and despite

*the fact that Nikki and Clay had emailed them that they didn't have
sex on first dates. That didn't stop Amy from asking Jack, "Do you
think we'll be fucking these people tonight?"*

*"We just might end up having a little sex," he said. Jack believed
the no-sex policy was a disclaimer in case they didn't like each
other; he assured Amy that the other couple would like them.*

*Amy wanted to arrive fashionably late for their date. They
arrived early, so they waited across the street from The Alley in
Carlsbad, California, and watched the club's front door. To their
shock, Clay and Nikki walked up, and right on time.*

*Jack kissed Nikki—it seemed like the thing to do. And he kissed
her again. Soon, Jack was sitting with Nikki and Amy with Clay. It
was fun confusing the waiter over who was with whom. Kiss. Drink.
Kiss. Dance. Kiss. Drink. Kiss. Dance. And it was time to leave.*

*Around 11 P.M., the foursome arrived at Jack and Amy's bed-
room, which Jack and Amy proudly called their entertainment
bedroom because it had a stereo, a TV, an eight-foot long couch,
and a queen-sized bed. Amy and Clay jumped in the bed. Jack and
Nikki piled on the couch. Nikki insisted on condoms. At that
moment, condoms became a rule for Jack and Amy, too. Jack and
Nikki had sex. Amy and Clay had sex. Amy and Nikki had sex,
while their husbands watched. Then Jack and Nikki had sex, while
Amy and Clay had sex.*

Two and a half hours later, Clay and Nikki said good night.

· · · · ·

By the time Jack, Amy, and I connected through Craigslist, they'd
had three dates with Clay and Nikki and had made plans to go to
Las Vegas with them.

"The wife is bi and I can dig that," Amy said. "Her husband is
very sweet, one of those sort of serious computer types but very
sexy."

Another reason Jack and Amy liked Clay and Nikki was because
they were committed to each other. "neither would do anything to

hurt the other and that takes out the danger and drama and just leaves the fun sex. and boy is it fun."

And boy, Jack and Amy were fun for me. I'd finally found a couple of swingers who were willing to talk to me in depth. Best of all, they were a safe eleven hundred miles away. To paraphrase Amy, it took out the danger and drama and just left the fun.

"we are pretty average looking," Amy wrote, "not fat, but not hot either, but you know what they say; it is all in the attitude. and we've got lots of that."

I'd heard that "it" was in the attitude, but I'd never comprehended that. At least not when it came to sex.

"you know the biggest problem with swinging is that you never can tell anyone about any of it. I was dying to tell someone about the cl husband, but you just can't do that. people just can't understand that don't swing. so it is kind of fun to talk about it."

I knew what she meant. Coyote had just emailed me a hug to help me through the day, but I couldn't tell my shrink about it because it would probably result in another scolding.

Amy couldn't talk about swinging at work. She feared it might cost her her job. She most definitely couldn't talk about it with her family. She was reared in a Christian home so conservative that she was not allowed to use the word "butt." Her mother never talked to her about sex. "she could not handle it at all." So when Amy gave up her virginity at age fifteen, she thought of herself as "slutty."

"even at church in the old days I would check out the guys and imagine who I would fuck. but I would feel guilty for thinking about it. crazy, huh????"

No.

Then again, when I was fifteen, I'd stare at the church ceiling and imagine myself swinging from one chandelier to the other, wondering if I'd make it or fall.

Crazy, huh????

Amy and Jack "used to be" Christians. "you know, the kind

that goes to bible study and stuff. we slowly burnt out on the scene.
the people (not all, but a lot) are really the worst type."

In their churchgoing days, Amy had been twenty pounds overweight and a stay-at-home mom who felt that the wealthy, slim,
professional Christians in their church looked down on them—a
financially struggling young couple. "It all just started to unravel.
we started to buy Playboys and then porno movies and over the
years just started to have fun. I don't feel like a Christian at all
anymore, and it has little to do with God. I went back to school,
got my degree, and just sort of progressed forward. I wonder if that
makes any sense to you. I don't know if I believe in God or not. I
think it is ok not to know. we have not been to church in 18 years."

· · · · ·

"I really don't consider myself bi," Amy continued, "but I have
had so much fun with the wife of our new friends with the guys
watching. . . . but I enjoy him (her husband) more. I just really like
men. I feel ok about being with a girl. really it is fun."

I wondered if the lady doth protest too much. Was that me
judging?

"I kissed a few girls in the hot tub . . . but with the new people
I really actually went down on her and likewise. it was different
and fun. she is sweet and very soft. really different than a guy, and
I think she likes me too."

Sweet and soft. I thought about that for a moment.

I wondered if sex with a woman was a way to have sex that was
tender, with boundaries that were respected, that wasn't scary and
physically painful.

As for Clay, Amy liked the way he flirted with her. "he is good
at complimenting and sweet talking, you know, stuff your husband
of 27 yrs doesn't need to say and it makes me feel really good about
myself. and best of all no strings attached. he does not love me. I
don't love him. it is just all for fun, sort of. it is hard to explain."

Makes me feel good about myself. No strings attached. He does not love me. I don't love him. Just fun.

No, it wasn't hard to explain. I understood completely.

· · · · ·

That night, Rose invited me for a visit. I was feeling a bit down due to my shrink's beratement—or at least what felt like a berating—that I didn't have enough fun in my life and a good enough support system. So instead of seeing my friend who had kissed me so sweetly so many, many months before, I printed out the Centers for Disease Control report "Sexual Behavior and Selected Health Measures," tossed my stuffed animals to the floor, and climbed into bed.

Beneath the lamplight I read, "Among females 15–44 years of age, 8 percent had never had sex, 7 percent had had sex with a male partner in their lives but not in the last 12 months."

I lay there and wondered what the stat was for women who'd gone without sex for ten years. Then again, I was over their age criteria, and when I'd been forty-four years old, I'd gone without sex for only four years.

Six percent of males, 15–44 years old, had had oral or anal sex with a man sometime in their lives, the report said. I thought that statistic was low, at least according to my research.

"Among females, 5.8 percent of teens and 4.8 percent of females 20–24 years of age had had both male and female partners in the last 12 months; percentages were lower at ages 25–44." That sounded reasonable.

Then I highlighted, "There is evidence, however, that certain diseases can be transmitted through oral sex, including gonorrhea, chlamydia, chancroid, and syphilis."

Hard swing, soft swing, it didn't matter—one was still at risk for a sexually transmitted infection.

I rolled over, turned out the light, and closed my eyes.

On Jack and Amy's second date with Clay and Nikki, in the hot tub, Nikki mounted Jack, without a condom. He waited awhile before asking, "Are we breaking one of your rules?"

She said yes but just kept right on sexing him.

"So, yeah, we think about STDs," Jack wrote me, "but what are you going to do. It all happens like a load of bricks falling on you. It's a little hard to keep your head straight."

· · · · ·

Five days later, I clicked on Craigslist's casual encounters in New York City and read, "Suit and Tie guy with an edge looking for cpl in their 50's—m4mw—42." I liked that phrase—"Suit and Tie guy."

"Would you consider talking to me about the lifestyle?" I typed and hit send.

"Discretion would be required. What did you have in mind?" He signed an initial only.

I explained that I didn't have to know his real name, we could start out by email, and if he eventually wanted to move on to phone, we could, but we didn't have to.

By the next day, he asked me to call him Neil and recommended that I sign up with swappernet.com to meet "real couples" who swing. "Meet and greets as they are called, are quite common. Just going out and meeting people to see if you click." Neil thought those groups were full of bicurious women who enjoyed being with other bicurious women and "Gillette commercial–looking guys."

"And I just don't go for that shit," he wrote. "They're disco ball. I'm candlelight."

I wasn't sure what I was, though probably not disco ball. As I said, I don't dance.

About the time disco was giving way to Madonna, Neil met a woman with whom he had "a pretty hot" monogamous sex life. In fact, it was so good that they moved in together. Fifteen years into their relationship, she had a hysterectomy. "It was like turning off a light switch. She lost all interest."

Here we go again. I was so tired of hearing men rationalize their cheating by complaining that their wives had lost all sexual interest due to menopause or a hysterectomy. I guess I should finally admit that I've had a hysterectomy.

Neil's lover was forty-four at the time of hers; he was thirty-five. I was thirty-seven at the time of mine. And my hysterectomy had nothing to do with the demise of my desire for sex. It wasn't just life, family, Texas, work, lack of confidence, acne, and weight that killed it either. The men I met contributed, too—they wanted relationships. Marriage, even. One wanted kids. I wanted to say, "You're barking up the wrong tree, buddy." But I didn't. Instead, the next time he called, I told him about my bad day, because I knew that'd get rid of him. And it did. I never heard from him again.

After "intimate rejection after rejection," Neil slowly suggested to his partner that she get counseling and medical help. "And it just wasn't happening."

Neil then purchased a computer. "And all of a sudden in three weeks you've sunk to the seventh level of hell—because it's *there*." He ventured into a porn site "and those cookies in your computer are going out like people feeding geese at a public park." He got a spam email about a couples' party in Massachusetts, just two and a half hours away. "I asked if single guys were ever invited and the reply was yes. I went to the party, couldn't believe it and haven't turned back."

With that, Neil decided he'd rather talk on the phone. So late the next afternoon, I call him as he is walking his dog. On the record, Neil won't detail where he works except to say he is with a New York City–based nonprofit and labors a lot of hours doing a lot of good for a lot of people. Therefore, he doesn't have a lot of time to cultivate a long-term relationship, nor does he want one.

My kind of guy.

Neil claims he is no longer romantically involved with the hysterectomy woman, but he still owns property with her and she doesn't know about his sex life—it would hurt her.

And that brought us back to Neil's first swing party. It was held in a private home owned by an older couple—he in his sixties, she in her late forties—who supplemented their income with the parties. They had a hot tub and a swimming pool, and once darkness closed in, the partiers shed their clothes and dived in. Neil spotted a man sitting on the edge of the pool. Then he noticed that a woman was going down on the man. Neil couldn't believe it. Quickly, he became an active participant in the "freakishly common" lifestyle.

But Neil didn't place himself willy-nilly in the swing world. He target marketed. He observed that men in their mid-fifties would get a prescription for Viagra and then gently push or nag their wives into swinging. Their wives, in their late forties or early fifties, were classy, sophisticated, and, in Neil's assessment, horny all the time, which made me wonder about the accuracy of the menopause/hysterectomy factor that men so self-righteously blamed. According to Neil, these women have been with very few men or only their husbands, and their husbands are so busy chasing unobtainable young women that they aren't bothering to communicate with their wives.

That's where Neil turns on his charm. Needless to say, he'd always been a fan of older women. He loved talking with them. "And that's such a turn on to some women"—a man who asks them what they want to talk about and actually listens to what they have to say. Neil makes sure to speak their names. He listens. He learns. He has great conversations that provide an intimate edge, which puts the sex over the top, just like Rex said. Neil calls it "wow, insane" sex.

He insists he's not a predator. He doesn't want a woman to cheat on her husband. He's just found an opportunity and has turned it into a positive for all.

Some people may think what he does is morally objectionable, he admits. "My take on it is it's consenting adults and it's a mutually pleasurable thing. . . . I have no problems with what I enjoy and with what people I meet enjoy."

I had no problems with Neil either. He sent me a photograph of himself. In it, he was fully clothed, in fact, wearing dark slacks, a white shirt, and a dark bow tie, so that he looked a bit like a maestro, and he was leaning back in his office chair with his hands relaxed behind his head. He looked safe. And he looked nice.

■ ■ ■ ■ ■

And with that, I guess I should confess another truth.

As Frank the swing club owner said to me, "You know you've thought about it." I wasn't about to admit it to Frank, but I *had* thought about it. Not in a swing club—or even a party—scenario. Neither of those enticed me. But when I lived in L.A., my best friend and I were hanging out one night in her favorite Melrose Avenue bar, when two *gorgeous* guys started talking to us. Over the Ms. Pac-Man machine, they asked us to leave with them. I wanted to. I'll repeat—they were *gorgeous*. My friend said no. She whispered that it was weird that these men couldn't seem to decide which one of them wanted which one of us. One minute, guy #1 talked to me and guy #2 talked to her. The next minute, they switched—guy #2 talked to me and guy #1 talked to her. I thought they were being nice; I was used to men being nice to me to get to her. Once, a man came up to me in a bar and said he and all of his buddies thought I was terrific. I said, "Why?" They'd only known me an hour or two. He said, "Because we figure if you can hang out with that blond bombshell and still keep smiling, you must be great." So I just thought these two men were talking to me because they thought I was great in the sidekick/best friend sort of way. My best friend thought they were bisexuals looking to have sex with each other and both of us.

I was intrigued.

I kept my intrigue to myself.

My best friend and I kept playing Ms. Pac-Man. The two gorgeous men left. My friend was happy. I was bored. When I got home that night, the phone rang. It was the two gorgeous men. They wanted me to come join them. I wanted to. I *really* wanted to. But

it was the 1980s. Too often, gay men I knew mysteriously disappeared, only to reappear months later, emaciated and gray-skinned,
torn remnants of their former selves. Others never returned; I only
heard rumors of their deaths. I was scared—scared of AIDS . . .
and my best friend finding out what I'd done. I turned down the
two men. Part of me has always been grateful that I did. Part of me
has always regretted it.

Yes, I've thought about it.

Chapter 33

• • • • •

"Tell me the pros and cons of how swinging has affected your marriage, communication, sex lives, and self-esteems," I wrote Jack and Amy.

"it definitely affects me," Jack said. "i'm not totally happy all the time with amy hanging out and fucking clay, but my best balance on the deal is that i get to hang out with and have sex with nikki. you can't tell me that's not a weird way of looking at our marriage. i start looking at other people's marriages and trying to put our dating other couples in some kind of perspective. i think most guys want to do other girls anyway, in marriage, so guys are probably mentally swinging from the go. we just don't like our women having fun too. that's about the only thing i can make out of why i would not want amy doing what i do. . . . i'm resigned that we will probably be ok."

Resigned. That sounded scary to me.

Jack then compared swinging to an electric miter saw he owned. The saw didn't have a guard on it. "when i turn it on and the blade is humming along with no guard, it weirds my body out and i can actually feel where every part of my body is in relation to that blade.

my fingers, hands, arms, everything. it's kind of like that. [our] level of commitment is definitely brought to the surface, and you get to take a good hard look at it—often. there, that's one for the pro column. i don't know which column the rest of it goes in. communicating? we talk about swinging a lot. it's fun to talk about. . . . i realize someone could ask us if fun is worth risking our marriage, but i think we needed to shake it up somehow. . . . i think things have to be exactly even for this to work, and i realize that exactly even is ludicrous. right now i can feel myself being selfish and hoping if it's not equal that i get the more equal helping."

I was surprised. I'd expected Jack to say he loved every aspect of swinging.

Amy was surprised, too. But they'd seen Clay and Nikki for the past two Saturdays, and Amy wondered if that was maybe just too intimate for Jack, though she needed that intimacy. "it is a vulnerable position for a girl. you need to feel safe and not afraid of what the guy might do." With Clay, she knew what was coming, so she wasn't afraid of him, in any way. "that's worth a lot to a girl."

Yes, it is.

She repeated that Clay's attached to his wife and talks about her all the time. "so I don't feel like I'm getting in over my head."

That's why I liked married men.

She said swinging's good for one's self-esteem "when you are hooking up," but it's "a big downswing when someone does not respond to an email after you send a picture. can you imagine that???"

I stared at the photo Jack had attached. Amy's black knit, V-neck top dipped so low and scooped so wide that it revealed her ample cleavage and at least half of her tanned bosoms. My eyes were drawn next to her firm legs, as her skirt covered only their top quarter. Finally I noticed Jack, tall, slim, slightly balding, and casually dressed.

But what were their facial expressions? I don't recall. I couldn't stop staring at those breasts. I don't usually notice breasts. But these, my Lord, the cleavage was a natural gorge. Not looking at it would be like refusing to look at the Royal Gorge.

Amy admitted she and Jack didn't really know what they were doing when it came to swinging. They were still trying to figure it out. As proof, after she read Jack's email to me, she realized that their communication wasn't as good as she'd thought. But she didn't think either one of them wanted to give up swinging. "You just keep doing it cause it is like crack when it goes good."

· · · · ·

With Amy, Jack, and Neil—in fact, with all of my sex freaks—my research was like crack to me, especially when it was going good. And it was going very well. Out of the blue, I received an email from Phoebe and Phil, lifestyle friends of Neil's. Neil had given them my email address, and quickly I learned that Neil and Phoebe had thrown swing parties together. Specifically in room 314, what they called the DNA room, at a hotel in Connecticut. "If you went into that place with a light, the frigging place would be glowing," Neil said.

I laughed and groaned, as I thought about all the TV news stories I'd watched where reporters had gone into hotel rooms to shine UV lights on the bodily fluids left behind.

Phoebe gave me her cell phone number, along with the advisement "that phone talk of this kind is only done when the kids are not around," and she and Phil offered to meet in person, if I were ever in New York City.

I said let's start out with email.

Phoebe then emailed me profiles she and Phil had posted on swinger websites from New York City to Washington, D.C.

"We are discreet professionals by day, but when the moon comes up, and the candles are lit, we walk on the wild side," they wrote in one. I presumed Phoebe was the author of the lines that said they disliked "men who cum quickly and think that once they cum their duty has been served. This is about mutual satisfaction, folks, not just getting some guy off."

I liked her already.

"It is our desire (but not mandatory) that the female of the couple be happily bisexual. . . ." Phoebe was bi, Phil straight. "And always, of course, NO means NO." They were willing to begin with soft swing "and move forward for those who are at different levels. . . . Plus we do not mind being the 'dirty little friends' you get crazy with, in fact we don't mind at all."

Their ad specified that they were turned off by drunks and pretenders, as well as "directors," "judgmental egotists," and "those who would attempt to use their lifestyle activity as a method to provide emotional pain to their mate, rather than the mutually nurturing and shared enjoyment it should be. Anyone who would disrespect/disregard another's expressed boundaries or comfort level!! No pressures given or accepted."

It declared that they liked "a pretty face as much as the next person, BUT ultimately it is what is on the inside, a self-confidence, comfort in one's own skin, sense of humor and intelligence that will keep our attention. We enjoy getting with people who know what they want, and are not afraid to just let loose. If you are afraid of getting loud and sweaty then we will probably scare you off. LOL."

Based on that—their desire for self-confident partners who were comfortable in their own skin and not afraid to let loose—I certainly felt I'd be safe with Phoebe and Phil. Besides, they specifically stated that they didn't try to convert others into the lifestyle.

Methodically, they'd created different profiles "to attract different types of people at different times." Purposely, their Washington, D.C., profile had more of an edge: "We are a sexy couple who loves to fuck and I mean fuck. . . . Phoebe has a smooth waxed hot little pussy that can suck your cock dry. We love all kinds of sex and like it all types of way. . . . I am an anal queen who does both double

vaginal penetration and conventional DP [double penetration]. . . .
Ladies, he is long lasting and considerate—I can guarantee you will
be totally satisfied."

One thing that made me like Phil and Phoebe—besides Phoebe's
dislike for men who came quickly—was that an absolute must of
theirs was good teeth. Plus, they made me laugh: "We do not care
for women who are not clean shaven, or at the least very closely
trimmed. Our bag of toys does not include a weed whacker."

Lord, that had me howling.

"It is kind of funny to us that we are the same people in all
3 profiles, yet some that would be attracted to us after reading ONE
profile would be totally turned off reading one of the others,"
Phoebe wrote me. "We have in fact contacted the same people from
2 different profiles and they replied sorry you are not our type to
one and yeah, let's meet ASAP to the other, proving our little experiment."

· · · · ·

The following day, Phoebe, who was in her early forties, and Phil,
who was in his mid-thirties, sent me a joint email. In it, Phil
explained that he first heard about swinging when he was an officer
in the military. Several of his unit members swapped partners. Phil
claimed he had no interest in swinging then, even though he immediately went out and purchased a swingers magazine, as well as an
amateur swingers party video.

But when one of his girlfriends—and he'd had numerous long-
term relationships, though he'd always cheated (and had felt guilty
about it)—told him she was interested in swinging, Phil spilled the
news to one of his female coworkers, whom he was already seeing
on the side for "really intense 'booty calls.'" The coworker said she
could help—she thought his girlfriend was gorgeous. So one night
at a club, she whispered to Phil's girlfriend that she wanted to take
them both to bed. She did—that night.

According to Phil, all three of them loved the experience, and he decided that from then on he was going to be up front and tell all future girlfriends that he's a swinger.

Fortunately for him, his next girlfriend also liked to swing. And that's how Phil met Phoebe—at a private swing party.

· · · · ·

The first thing Phoebe told me was that she was in the middle of a divorce. In fact, she and her husband hadn't lived together for the past five years, but, according to her, their marriage had been "on a downward spiral" since shortly after the birth of their ten-year-old son. That's when their sex life became so boring that Phoebe "began to see it as a chore—like washing laundry. It was to the point where when we had sex, all I could think about is please let this be over soon."

To alleviate the boredom, Phoebe began visiting bisexual chat rooms, first as a voyeur, then participating in conversations. Phoebe next noted that she'd "dabbled" with girls in both high school and college. "Never even THOUGHT about mentioning this to my husband." She did mention it to a professional athlete she met in a chat room. "And so for my birthday that year, he got us a woman," after which, and at Phoebe's suggestion, she signed them up with a swinging website. "Phil and I actually started talking through one of those sites and then chatting online regularly for a year and a half or so before we ever met at that 'fateful' party."

Only when I asked Phoebe and Phil if anyone at their work knew they were swingers did Phil disclose that he was still in the military. Admittedly, there's "an entire military [swinging] subculture." Indeed, many in the lifestyle say swinging began in the air force. Still, Phil believes that if his participation was made public, it would damage his career. "I have a graduate level clinical psychology back[ground], with research/clinical sex therapy, and our society is horrible at facing the sexual sides of our lives."

But when Phil added, "Where else can a factory worker from PA meet a neurosurgeon at a party thrown by someone who has connections to the Gotti family," I thought that if swinging couldn't help one's career, it sure could make life interesting.

"I have met the Consul General of a European country and his wife," Phoebe said. "Have been to their Central Park West apartment. Now this man is in his 60s, and let me tell you HE does have some really strange fetishes."

Phoebe—who asserted that she consummated nearly all of her high school and college male friendships and gave a blowjob to the owner of an international clothing firm "in the back of his Rolls Royce as his driver was going down 5th Avenue," as well as to a doctor who worked at the hospital where she's a nurse (both blow-jobs with the help of her sister)—grew up in a traditional American family. Her parents married, never cheated, never divorced, and her mother turned scarlet at the mention of sex.

Phil's childhood, which included years in Europe, was the complete opposite. His grandfather and father openly had mistresses. His parents' marriage ended in divorce, but Phil emphatically stated that his father's affairs had nothing to do with that. "He decided to get drunk and take a swing at my mom and she drew the line there." Besides, his mother had her own history of being "the other woman," he said. "So I am simply carrying on the family tradition with an open sexuality."

"Thank you for this," I responded, "and for clarifying things. I was under the impression that y'all were married to each other." And I didn't say much else about their meticulous five-page email. I think I was a bit upset, angry, and disappointed that they were swing partners with each other rather than with their own spouses. Yes, I eventually discovered that Phil was married, too. I had no right or reason to have those feelings, but time and again I'd been told that swinging was about honesty and that it wasn't cheating if the spouse knew and was involved. Yet here Phil and Phoebe were, and it seemed to me what they were doing was just plain ole, regular cheating, not swinging.

Two days later, and at my request, Phoebe sent me another long email explaining her marriage. According to her, her husband changed from a kind, generous, funny, and great friend to a violent man with alcohol and gambling problems. Their divorce would be final by the end of the year.

Although she and Phil had an immediate online rapport, and she found herself being "fairly open" with him about "most things," when they first met, she led him to believe she was married to the pro athlete. Phil still believed that when he and Phoebe began meeting on the sly. Soon, though, she confessed her true marital status.

"I have been able to say things to him about my life, good and bad, that I have never said to ANYone else, even my sister who I love dearly. I felt I could say things to Phil without fear of ridicule or condemnation, or his saying I told you so.

"To take from the Rod Stewart song, 'you're in my heart.' He really is my lover, my best friend and 'til the day I die, he will be in my heart and in my soul.

"Then he has this great big . . .

"BRAIN.

"betcha thought I was going to say something else, didn't you???

"Well there is THAT too, but. . . . .

"He is also very enigmatic, and that air of mystery makes him all the more appealing. Besides that he is kinda cute. LOL.

"This is all without mentioning the sex.

"He is a practitioner in Tantra and let me tell you, if you have never experienced Tantric sex, then you have never felt worshipped. Sex has become like a religious experience and I say that because the man can make me see God, and more often than not the intensity moves me to tears. Who KNEW that there are actually men who put the woman's pleasure before theirs?? Was all new to me. I never knew I could be multi and I mean MULTI orgasmic.

"I am content for the first time in a very long time. The man gives me peace of mind . . . and an almost giddy sense of joy."

· · · · · ·

Phil's wife knew about Phoebe. They'd had a threesome. But his wife didn't know that Phoebe was in love with Phil and that Phil and Phoebe considered each other soul mates.

Phoebe explained that one can "love and share an intimate relationship with more than one person." She knew that Phil loved her. He told her that. "Do not get me wrong," she said, "we did not start out thinking that this relationship would take off the way it did. But we are where we are, and that is all there is to it."

Phoebe even chatted online with Phil's wife. At first, she felt "a bit guilty." Then she told herself, "You know what? I do not care."

But I wanted her to care. "Sisters" in the femininehood were supposed to support each other rather than hurt each other. That's what the 1960s and '70s had been all about. And I was a child of the '60s and '70s. In fact, that's one of the two reasons I'd stopped sleeping with married men—I didn't want to hurt their wives, my "sisters."

"I would never tell her, hey, I love your husband and we have had this really intense secret heavy duty relationship for 3 yrs.," Phoebe said.

Then there were the children. Phil was a new father. I'd once had a secretary who told me she and her father were, oh, so close, until she learned he was cheating on her mother. That destroyed her relationship with him.

That's the second reason I'd stopped sleeping with married men. And when I did, my sex life basically ended.

"It would serve no good purpose to any of us. In that regard, Phil and I decided long ago that if the opportunity came up, however remote it might be, that we could all play together, I would politely decline, as I feel that the connection between Phil and I is too obvious and it would be like a blazing beacon to her that there is something deeper going on. I respect her too much for that."

Phoebe further pointed out that she and Phil were in different stages of their lives. "And our age difference has a bit to do with that of course." But she stressed again that their relationship was more than the lifestyle and even more than sex. "I can say that when I am old and gray and sex is a far away memory I will still love this man all the same, will until the day I die. Listen not only would I trust him with MY life but I would trust him with the lives of each and every one of my kids."

Though Phoebe didn't use the word poly, to me it was obvious that they had a polyamorous relationship—with the exception of the "honesty with all involved" part—namely his wife. And, I guess, for them it worked. And I guess I had to respect that.

Chapter 34

· · · · ·

Jack and Amy sat in their car downing whiskey shooters trying to gather the confidence and courage to walk into the swing club. It was a private house—large, comfortable, and neat, though not outstanding in its 1980s curb appeal—in a residential neighborhood of San Diego. Twice a month the home was transformed into a members only, couples only sex club for partner swapping. Already, Jack and Amy had submitted their application for membership, been interviewed, and accepted.

Nonetheless, at seven o'clock on this fall Saturday evening, it was one more shot of whiskey courage before they stepped out of their car and introduced themselves to Ken and Heather. Ken and Heather were another pair of first timers, and like Jack and Amy, they'd arrived early for new member orientation.

As the four of them walked up the long, curving front drive, they nonchalantly checked one another out. Amy didn't even consider flirting with Ken and Heather. They appeared to be beautiful people in their thirties. She thought they'd be looking for playmates their own age. Her middle-aged breasts nearly overflowed her bra top. A short, fringed denim and plaid skirt accentuated her strong *legs. Newly manicured toes peeked out of her clear high heels. Jack wore a long-sleeved Western shirt, Levi's jeans, and black cowboy boots. The club's theme for the night—and there was always a theme—was fun times "down on the farm."*

They gave their names to the volunteer who greeted them and guarded the front door. Just inside, another volunteer flipped through the pages of her new members' guest list. Jack's and Amy's names weren't there. Neither was their new members' card. "Whatever," the volunteer said, then checked their driver's licenses, had them sign a release swearing they weren't carrying drugs and weren't law enforcement or news media, and sent them to orientation.

A husband-and-wife team—she wearing see-through lingerie—toured them through the home. After Jack got over the shock of the see-through lingerie, he assessed the house. Immaculate, good paint job, not a thing broken. By then, they stood in a room decorated with a wall of beds—two rows of beds, one on top of the other, each row divided by solid walls into three large cubbyholes, like giant, built-in shoe shelves. Every cubbyhole contained a full-sized mattress covered with a white sheet and a white curtain draped to the side.

"Don't open closed curtains," they were warned. "They're for privacy."

Aluminum stepladders leaned against the beds, since it was a four-foot climb up to the second row. Cups full of condoms and lubricant were attached to each headboard. The guides pointed out the condoms and encouraged their use. A bastion of responsibility, Jack thought.

"If you need to spend the night, we'll put a nameplate on one of the cubbies for you so that you know where you can stay," they were told. But they were also advised that they weren't supposed to spend the night—that was only an option if they were too intoxicated to drive. And if they did stay, "You can help clean up in the morning."

In a second bedroom, three king-sized beds were lined side by side. They were directed not to use the whole bed, so that "others can use the unused half." A third bedroom had two more cubby-holes, a castle-like décor, and manacles hanging from the wall for light bondage play. A fourth bedroom had two queen-sized beds. Again, they were cautioned to use only half the bed, in order to leave room for others—and to use condoms. Finally, they were led into a fifth bedroom with two king-sized beds, for a total of fifteen beds throughout.

Outside, there was a pool and a hot tub. Inside, there was a "down on the farm" buffet—ribs, chicken fried steak, macaroni and cheese, potatoes, corn, green beans covered in bacon, raw vegetables, dips, and Crock-Pots warming chicken wings and sausages. Jack and Amy were handed plates and plastic forks and ate, while soaking in every detail. There were at least twenty volunteers, each wearing a name tag, all doing the cooking and the cleaning, all friendly and inviting. There were short skirts, short shorts, low-cut blouses, see-through blouses, and teddies.

Finally, nearly a dozen new couples were ushered onto the dance floor, where they were given the house rules one more time. "No drugs. Don't even use Viagra unless you're used to it."

By 11 P.M., women with their tops down, tops up, and tops off crowded the dance floor. But Jack wasn't sure what to do. He looked around. He reached for Amy's hand, led her onto the wood floor, lifted her short skirt, and worked her panties. Immediately, a couple began flirting with them—Brad, an architect, and his ex-wife Faith. The divorced couple still partied together but only in separate rooms. Jack and Faith left to find a cubbyhole, while Amy and Brad found their own bed.

"You have to put on a condom," Amy insisted, as she and Brad touched.

Brad argued that he'd had a vasectomy.

"I don't want to explain to Jack why we didn't use a condom," she coaxed.

Reluctantly, Brad rolled one on.

· · · · ·

"*You don't really need one," Faith said as Jack reached for the condom bowl. "Just put your penis in a little bit." Jack put his penis in just a little bit, as they discussed the pros and cons of condoms. "I don't really like the way they feel," Faith said.*

Makes sense to me, *Jack thought. She felt so good around him. Besides, he, too, had had a vasectomy. He moved deep inside of Faith and there was no pulling out before he came.*

· · · · ·

Twenty minutes later, Amy and the architect were finished. She checked on Jack. He was still busy with Faith, so Amy meandered into the living room, where she watched a woman perform oral sex on men who passed through the room. Ken, the thirty-something beautiful newcomer, joined Amy. He teased her that she had on panties. She whipped them off and socked them on his head. He groped under her skirt. Then he ripped off her shirt. "Let's go dance," he said.

But Amy wanted to check on Jack again. He was still occupied with Faith, so Amy stepped onto the dance floor with Ken, where they took off the rest of their clothes, then kissed. And she sucked him.

"Let's go to a room," Ken said.

"I thought you were dancing," his wife interrupted.

Heather, Ken, and Amy went to a room. As Amy licked the young wife, she noticed that rings pierced both of Heather's nipples and her clitoris. And when it came time for Ken and Amy to have intercourse, he refused to wear a condom.

"I don't want to get pregnant," Amy claimed. She flirted, "You look like you would be dangerous in that respect." Ken had the hard body of a marine, which he was.

He put on a condom, but as soon as he was inside Amy he lost his erection. They agreed to stick to oral sex, tossed the condom, and rolled into the 69 position. Ken's penis was engorged in Amy's mouth when Jack found them. He threw off his clothes and piled in.

"amy is SUCH a slut. i am such a perv," Jack emailed me afterward.

"Yes, it is true. I am a big slut," Amy giddily chimed in. "Can't wait to go back."

• • • • •

That night, I couldn't sleep. My body ached with tension. At 3 A.M., I got up and checked to see if Jack had sent me another email. Another one didn't arrive until the following afternoon.

"i'd like to make a comment on the use of condoms in swing clubs. people don't use them," Jack said. "i've come to believe that condom use is an endangered species at these places. . . . amy and i are going to have to come to some agreement about using condoms or we're going to be a statistic pretty soon. but when i'm looking at faith and she wants me to enter her just a little . . . now, on monday, i'm thinking maybe i should have used that condom."

He reminded me that Nikki always used a condom, except when she was in the hot tub. "so let's review," he said. "everyone we've been with so far uses condoms, except when they think a condom isn't going to feel good or getting the condom is inconvenient. houston, i think we have a problem."

Yes.

• • • • •

According to the CDC data that I went to bed with seemingly each night, HIV/AIDS cases were increasing in those over age forty-five and among whites, males, heterosexuals, and men who had sex with men, which covered so many of my sources. But no one except me seemed concerned about condoms and STDs.

I'd talked to Phoebe and Phil about this, too. They were "absolute condom users," Phoebe insisted. Then again, there was a couple they frequently played with and they didn't use condoms with them. In fact, Phil admitted he and Phoebe were condom users only 95 percent of the time and they never used them during oral sex. I don't think I had a single source who used condoms during oral sex.

Once again I thought about all the diseases one can get through unprotected oral sex—HPV, gonorrhea, chlamydia, syphilis, cancer of the throat and mouth, herpes, HIV.

"I don't want you to jump to the wrong conclusion," Phoebe had insisted during one of several phone conversations we'd had. "We know a lot of people." Hundreds of swingers. "[But] we have a select few that we've actually played with. So it's not like we're out having major, major random acts of sex with everybody we meet. . . ."

I wanted to believe her. But I also knew it didn't take hundreds. It took one.

It was enough to stress a single Southern Baptist woman into celibacy.

Chapter 35

•••••

Jack was stressed about their upcoming trip to Vegas with Clay and Nikki. Nikki had told him that the only reason they were swinging was to make Clay happy. Clay had told Amy that the only reason they were swinging was to make Nikki happy. "and i have gotten a little bent out of shape at clay for emailing amy so often about the vegas trip. i told amy it was starting to look like the clay and amy show. . . ."

What Jack and Amy didn't know was that often when they were having problems due to swinging, I'd email Phil and Phoebe about them. I don't mean I'd say, hey, I know these swingers in San Diego named Jack and Amy, and they're . . . I was (sometimes) a bit more subtle. For example, when Jack had first mentioned his jealousy issues, I'd emailed Phil and Phoebe about their own relationship, asking them how and when it had become polyamorous and if moving from swinging to a polyamory was typical in the swing community.

Phil thought all lifestylers who slept with a friend they cared about and "put no limits on the love between them" were practicing a type of polyamory. He also believed that love was something that should be shared, whatever form it took. But he stated that poly-amory wasn't typical in the swinging lifestyle. "I have known sev-eral couples who split up because one partner develops a crush on another partner from another couple. This is typically the guy and the guy will try to leave his family because he develops a crush on someone."

I thought about Clay.

"The main thing is being honest with your partner."

I thought about Jack.

"this whole swinging thing is like walking on shaky ground," Jack said, "but i will tell you that amy and i have had to get to the root of my mental distress, jealousy issues and i'm sure other crap that has drifted to the surface. . . . i think usually i would just be angry for awhile and let time heal the wound. but so much emo-tional material comes so fast, not to deal with it would be corrosive to our relationship." So at least they were talking about it, he said. "now if you happen to spot a root problem here, just chime right in. we are laying everything out as it happens and we're not editing."

I just told them to enjoy Vegas . . . and I wished I could silently follow them, observing them.

But Vegas turned out to be a "train wreck," to use Jack's termi-nology. Nikki got jealous of Amy. Nikki and Clay had a fight about it. Amy and Jack did, too. Jack harangued Amy that she and Clay looked and acted like they were dating, thanks to all of the emails and instant messages they exchanged. "i told amy that one of these days i would run across a girl and that it would appear like i liked her more than amy. better looking, better personality, better all the way around. it's inevitable."

That didn't sound good to me.

"i told her at some point we would have a big problem in our relationship because of who knows what's coming. . . . I think it never really sank in for amy until she got the email that nikki was having the jealousy problem."

Then Nikki and Clay dumped Amy and Jack.

Jack told me, "so wtf!" Amy told me she'd always known things were going to end badly with Clay and Nikki. "And to tell you the truth, I couldn't wait. It was just so fun and crazy and wrong and different. I couldn't help myself."

The problem was music. She and Clay had started talking about music and they'd connected through that. "And even though it is a harmless connection, it still was a connection outside of the swinging sex deal, and it threw the whole deal out of whack," Amy said. "but now I look back and think any kind of connection besides just plain ole sex is a problem, because sex is easy and straight forward but it is all the other stuff that turns sex into a relationship."

So Jack told me that from now on Amy was going to communicate only with their female partners, "regardless of who is pushing the deal, out of sight."

"I will miss hanging with them," Amy said, "but must press on and see what the next chapter brings. No regrets."

The next chapter.

· · · · ·

I had mixed emotions when thinking about the next chapter for me. While Phil was deployed overseas, Phoebe and I were communicating regularly. I don't mean heavy-duty, emotional emails like I was exchanging with Jack and Amy. There were just those few phone calls and many quickie notes that made me laugh—comical stories about Neil and his swing life, whacky stories about the parties they'd thrown, exchanges about the pains and benefits of Brazilian wax jobs, and jokes about a DNA party they allegedly planned on throwing for me. In the course of one of our phone conversations, she'd blurted, "We're going to Vegas in April. You wanna make a reservation?"

"I might have to," I laughed.

The next day, she emailed me that she was planning to meet a single, bisexual female—"the ever elusive 'unicorn,' (yes that is what they are known as in the swing world in that they are THAT rare)"—in hopes that the woman would become a regular player with her and Phil.

She emailed me again later that day, promising to invite an eclectic mix to the DNA party they now seriously planned on throwing for me. "And you have an open invite should you dare, heeheeeee."

I knew the dare didn't mean showing up at the party. It meant participating.

"Oh . . . we know I want to dare . . . via observation, LOL," I joked back. I would be there, I said, "clothes on."

"Never say never regarding playing," she returned. "We have made converts out of harder cases than you perceive yourself to be."

I simply signed my next email "Suzy—your very own uptight, white journalist."

I thought that said everything that needed to be said—I was a journalist doing her job; I would not be participating other than watching and taking notes. Besides, I didn't take her conversion statement seriously, since I had it in writing—via their swinger profile—that they didn't try to convert others into the lifestyle.

Hanging in the back of my mind, though, was her search for a unicorn.

So to ensure that Phoebe understood unquestionably that I would *not* participate, I explained that if I joined in the sex, my book would read like every other book out there on swinging. "What would make mine different," I said, "would be not participating. That way I could be totally objective."

I'm guessing my shrink would think I'd already lost objectivity with Phoebe. When Phoebe had told me she and Phil planned on joining the mile high club on their trip to Vegas, I'd joked, "I think I'd be more into oral sex under a blanket. Oops, I didn't say that. Gotta get my reporter hat back on."

And I don't care what my shrink would say, that wasn't flirtation. It was me being relaxed with a sex freak/source who liked to laugh and crack jokes. So when I specifically told Phoebe that I would not be participating, I also said, "Does that work for you?"

Then I joked again, "Besides, you don't even know what I look like."
And I inserted one of those stupid smiley face icons.

Of course, like so many of my other sources, Phoebe went online
and found a photograph of me. She thought that was only fair since
she'd sent me pictures of them. In Phil's photo, he simply looked
like a dark-complected man with a kohl moustache and goatee and
a buzz cut that made his ears stand out from his head. Phoebe's
picture recalled 1960s Hollywood glamour, as though she hung out
with Robert Wagner and Natalie Wood. Her shoulder-length,
bleached blond hair was straight and well cut. Hot pink glossed lips
were primly pursed into a smile, and mirrored sunglasses masked
a tanned face punctuated with a Peggy Lee–like beauty mark. In
fact, she reminded me of Peggy Lee.

I'd like to point out, though, that I wasn't communicating solely
with Phoebe just because Phil was overseas. Apparently, female-
to-female communication only was one of their rules, although
they'd never told me that. The one time I'd talked on the phone to
Phil, Phoebe had been on the phone with us. All of my queries to
Phil had gone through Phoebe. Even most of my communication
with Neil was going through Phoebe.

But with Jack and Amy, the majority of our communication was
through Jack.

Right then, Jack was telling me that they were beginning to
reconnect sexually with their neighbors, the ones who drank too
much. "come on, suzy," he wrote, "shake your head. we're out of
our minds, aren't we?"

I couldn't leave it at just that, though. I had to know more. Was
he still jealous of Amy and Clay? How did he feel about Amy going
down on women? How did he feel their marriage was holding up?

And Jack was willing to tell me. "am i jealous of them," he said.
"no. . . . i just have to talk it over with myself often." He didn't get
jealous either when Amy was with other women. "the whole thing
for a guy is pretty exhausting." In fact, letting Amy take over with
another woman was a "nice break" for him. "it's pretty cool just

sitting back and catching my breath. . . . i don't even feel compelled to watch. . . . i laugh to myself when guys talk three-way."

Amy had even started thinking of herself as bisexual.

Were Jack's and my constant emails becoming like Clay and Amy's? We'd been trading them for three hours in a single day. For me, I was doing my job. That's all. And I knew Amy read everything Jack wrote me. Still, I did ponder Jack's and my connection, as he discussed how their marriage was holding up.

"i've never experienced this depth of angst in 27 years [of marriage]," he said, "so maybe we're finally getting to know each other. i think that's why i'm not bitterly jealous (yet). if we end up breaking up it might be because we decided one of us really doesn't like the other person now that we're introduced. i don't think anybody really knows how secure their marriage is. about us breaking up, we decided years ago the person who initiates the break has to take the kids."

And I laughed.

Chapter 36

·····

"How was Halloween?" I wrote Jack and Amy. They'd celebrated the haunted weekend with a return trip to the swing club.

Jack answered a day later saying the joke may have been on them, though he'd have to tell me later—Amy couldn't stand to talk about it yet. "be patient."

Days passed before I heard from him again. Halloween hadn't been good—rejection by the girl he wanted, soft swing only with a woman who didn't shave anywhere, while great, full-throttle sex was going on in the bed next to him with much better-looking women. Everything wasn't perfect in swingerville, he said, especially since he couldn't stop replaying the rejection memories.

Then Jack rubbed his tongue along the inside of his lip, and his tongue bumped over something. He stared into the mirror, pulled out his lip, and looked. There was a tiny bubble—3/32 of an inch in size and an inch down his lip, toward his gums.

His tongue kept bumping over it, and each time it did, he was convinced he had herpes of the mouth. Jack popped the bubble, put some oil and oregano on it, and pronounced it well. But it came back. He repeated his treatment. That time the bubble didn't return, but a tiny bit of hardness replaced it. He grabbed a utility knife, jerked out the razor, and carved off the bump.

With that, Jack got on the Internet, researched herpes, and diagnosed himself disease-free. Despite his pronouncement, Jack wasn't all that sure. He was going to see a doctor. "add that into the mix," he wrote. And he wasn't speaking to Amy.

But as the week progressed, Jack began to calm. If he were confident that he and Amy were doing everything they could to protect themselves from sexually transmitted infections and if he could protect himself emotionally, he believed he could see swinging "as just being fun."

I didn't know how Amy felt. I couldn't get a response from her. I begged her for information. She eventually wrote, "Just need some time to piece it all together. God, life is complicated."

Amy was so silent that I feared someone had slipped a drug into her drink or hadn't stopped when she'd said no. I also feared her silence indicated she was angry with me about something.

That wasn't it.

"I went silent because something weird happened," she wrote, eight days before Thanksgiving. While riding her bicycle and then while having sex with Jack, she'd felt pain in what she called her "undercarriage." She went to her doctor, who thought Amy had a yeast infection. Then the doctor asked, "You are married, right? Just one sex partner, right?"

"So I had to tell her that well no there were a few dudes and she said oh well then it might be herpie. She called it 'Herpie.'"

Amy was swabbed "for every std known to man" and given medication for both a yeast infection and herpes. "In the depths of despair," she waited a week for her lab results. When she returned to the doctor's office, Amy told herself, *Whatever happens, I brought it on myself, I just have to live with it*. Finally, the doctor informed her that she didn't have herpes or any other STD, just a bad yeast infection and a bacterial infection.

"So now I feel like I fooled fate. out-smarted Herpie. now

what???? keep going??? get out while we can???? make a bunch of rules like Clay & Nikki???? Change our hunting grounds from the clubs to just more off the cuff casual stuff at bars and stuff. . . . Jack asked me tonight if I am surprised every time I read email and there is nothing there from Clay & Nikki. and yeah it is hard. but not surprising. . . . I miss the dates and having fun out knowing that later we would all end up together fucking in our bed and on the couch in our room. you don't get that very much in this world. most people are not that open-minded. I think they will be hard to replace. I could be wrong. God knows I am wrong a lot. But I would be a big fat liar if I said I did not miss them. . . . the final word on the subject, I am sad. but I love Jack. really. in a way I can't explain. he turns me on in about 2 seconds and he can be so sweet. still makes my heart pound in my chest when he touches me unexpectedly. do you know what I mean???? the other day we were on our front sidewalk talking to a neighbor and Jack put his arm around me and I almost had a heart attack. pretty good for 27 yrs. I don't think anyone ever in my life would be able to do that for me. I am hooked and in the boat. anyway, yea, no 'herpie.'"

And, dear reader, I know you already know what I'm about to say—no, I didn't understand what Amy meant about someone making her heart pound. By now, you know me better than my sources do . . . perhaps better than I know myself. . . .

• • • • •

But my heart began to pound in a very different way as the holidays approached. The day before Thanksgiving, I learned that my mother had a growth on one of her kidneys. Presumably, it was cancer. "I always wish you believed in God," I wrote Rose, "but, damn, at times like this, I really wish it."

I wanted, I needed, prayers for my family. I didn't know what I'd do without my mother. She was my thorn, and she was my rock. I couldn't concentrate on work, but for some strange reason—I guess it was a way to distract myself—I could still think on sex. Or maybe it was because Rose had just broken up with her boyfriend. Or maybe it was because Rose had reminded me that I'd told her I had a sex drive. That seemed a *very* long time ago.

"I think I said that last August when I'd lost a couple of pounds and had gotten a little sun and was hopeful that I was going to continue on the weight loss," I wrote her. "Instead, I gained back those pounds plus some and have returned to my sushi white pallor. Self-confidence, sexually and work-wise, is very low."

When I stood before the mirror, I saw an acne-faced, fifty-year-old female with a protruding white belly and bulbous thighs.

"I just can't imagine anyone being attracted to me. When I got my hair cut a few weeks ago, I was stunned when someone who was watching me get the cut said something about how I was so 'cute.' I just can't imagine.

"But I sometimes wonder if I had a couple of drinks in me and someone attractive touched me that I'd be all over them. I know the night I was drinking with the jazz cowboy that I certainly wanted to do some serious kissing.

"I don't know. I just don't know. I guess what I'm saying is that I can't imagine you ever being attracted to me or desiring me sexually. But if you ever want to touch me, well, don't do it unless you at least want some serious kissing, because I don't know how I'll respond. I'll either be all over you or sitting in a corner shaking, saying get away 'cause I'd hate for you to be grossed out by my appearance. And more than likely, you wouldn't want either reaction."

I guess what I was really saying was that like so many of my sex freaks, I was lonely and hurting.

God, I hate it when I get all honest.

Rose didn't reply.

. . . . .

Still, to be heartfelt and truthful with one of my dearest friends was one thing; to be honest with my sex freaks was another.

I'd emailed Phoebe and Phil a multitude of questions about

their relationship. After answering my queries, Phil wrote, "Since
we are 100% honest, now it is your turn." He wanted to know
what so sparked my interest in the lifestyle that I'd want to write
about it. "Remember," he said, "I have an extensive history in sex
therapy." He wondered if I was curious about what made them tick
and how a person's sexuality made them do things out of the ordinary.

"Have you been turned on by what some people have told you??

"Can you see yourself in a lifestyle relationship? Or does jealousy
get the best of you??"

"Whether or not you choose to respond to them is your choice,"
Phoebe said, "but we are curious."

My one-year "anniversary" of researching Americans' alternative sex habits was just one week away. After my early goof-ups, at
least according to my shrink and my shrink friend, I thought I'd
done a pretty decent job of keeping my thoughts, feelings, and life
private from my sex freaks. Of course, some of them, when I'd
refused to answer their questions about me, had refused to answer
any more of my questions. But I planned on communicating with
Phil and Phoebe for a very long time. And, as I once again stared
out my office door to the dark winter leaves of the live oak trees,
maybe I was just tired and vulnerable. I know I was discombobulated by my mother's health news.

So, yes, I answered, I was always curious about what made
anyone tick and what made someone do things out of the ordinary,
whether it was sex or murder or becoming a rock star. That was an
easy question.

I repeated that I was sick of true crime, emotionally beaten up
by it, and wanted to laugh again. I told Phil that my literary agent
had come up with the sex idea, that I saw it as my way out of true
crime, and I mentioned how I'd been hesitant to do the book. "Sex
just isn't that big of a deal in my life." I guess at that point in time
that was a lie, since it had consumed my life for nearly a year. "But

writers are supposed to write about the things that might be a psychological issue for them. I'm guessing that sex would fill that bill."

What an understatement.

And, yes, I admitted that what people told me sometimes turned me on. "A shrink friend tells me I shouldn't admit this to my sources. . . ."

I'm not sure whether that confession was a sign that I was progressing—that I was making my own decisions rather than relying on someone else—or that I was regressing and not following wise advice. I have a feeling it was a bit of both, and a lot of rebellion.

Could I see myself in the lifestyle? That question was moot, I said. I still had no desire to do relationships. And as for marriage, I still believed it ended in death or divorce, so why bother?

As usual, I described myself to Phil and Phoebe as boring—in fact, as "terribly, terribly boring."

"We, my dear," Phoebe wrote back, "are going to try like hell to change the perception you have of yourself. LOL."

The day after my fifty-first birthday, I sat at my computer, placed my fingers on the keyboard, and yelled, "Do it!" I emailed Neil and asked him to escort me to a New York City swing club. We'd go the same weekend Phoebe and Phil planned to throw their DNA room party just for me. I don't mean just for me in that the three of us would have sex. I mean they'd invite some swingers to a party, and I'd watch.

But you might ask why—after all the people who had invited me to swing parties, to watch them masturbate, to watch them have sex—why did I say yes to Phoebe and Phil and now ask Neil to take me to a swing club.

I asked Neil because he was the only single, swinging male who hadn't been overtly sexual and pushy with me. I said yes to Neil because, though he and Phoebe threw swing parties together, they'd never had sex together. That meant he could accept no. And I trusted him because I trusted Phoebe and Phil. In addition to our phone calls, Phoebe and I had traded literally hundreds of emails.

When I'd learned about my mother's illness, Phoebe—along with Coyote—had said prayers for her. When I'd learned that my mother's doctor had said let's just watch the tumor for a while, Phoebe—and Coyote—had wanted to know that. In fact, though Phoebe had said she wasn't very religious, she repeatedly mentioned prayer and God to me. Specifically, she prayed for the children she took care of. That touched me.

Then Phil sent me a note through Phoebe: "Make sure you tell her that our friendship is paramount . . . and the sexual aspect of it is a great bonus that brings us closer together."

That impressed me.

Phoebe added, "He listened to me talk about work, how I cry over kids that died on me, things that MATTERED to me mattered to him."

I liked these people.

And I liked the way they were looking out for me. Again, through Phoebe, Phil emailed, "Suzy, we just want to let you know that if you are planning on losing your swinging virginity, make sure you and Neil have discussed the parameters in which you both agree to play. It can be a terribly awkward moment to be in a room and one partner is not going to 'take one for the team.' So just talk about what you are willing to do before it gets to that situation. With everyone being naked some people may be a little more pushy towards having sex. I have been in a similar situation and people feel as though they can take certain liberties."

Is that why my aunt, the church secretary, had told me she didn't want me going to New York? Why she'd wanted to know what I could learn about these people in person that I couldn't learn over the phone? After all, I hadn't revealed to my family that I was going to a swing club. I was only going to New York to interview people, which was true, too.

Also true was that I *was* nervous about the trip. So nervous that

I wanted a safe female friend to accompany me. I asked Rose to go with me. She said no. I asked Lola to go with me. She said no. I begged and begged Phoebe and Phil to join Neil and me at the swing club. They refused.

So finally I emailed Neil and asked him what a voyeuristic prude would wear to a swing club.

He replied, "A nervous smile and a chastity belt perhaps?"

Through Neil and Phoebe, as well as my online research, I knew many lifestylers considered the club we were going to to be Manhattan's lowest end swing club. I'd heard complaints that only old, overweight, out-of-shape men and women frequented it. Good, I wouldn't feel out of place. I'd heard there were dirty sheets on its mattresses and God knows what on its dirty floors. *Oh, Lord.* Neil suggested I bring flip-flops to wear.

I knew—again through my online research—that the club's rules stated that one could be dressed in the lounge area but had to "disrobe" to go upstairs or into the "mat room." In other words, one had to get naked to see the action, which is what I was going to see. *Oh, Lord.* But I also knew one *could* wear a towel, which the club provided. I hoped they were beach towels and not hand towels.

Neil assured me they weren't beach towels. *Oh, Lord.*

Though I had a nervous smile, I didn't have a chastity belt, so I emailed Phoebe, "What do I wear? My preference would be a tent . . . but I guess hiding behind a lot of cloth isn't really appropriate."

She replied that the club "gets you naked as soon as you walk thru the locker room."

Oh, geez.

Then, as if I weren't nervous enough, she had to add, "AND we try to get people naked right off the bat as well. Wear whatever you're comfortable in."

I asked if I could wear flannel jammies. "I'd feel comfortable in that."

She told me I could wear a silky robe or lingerie as long as it wasn't ratty, cotton, white, or beige.

I was up shit creek.

On January 19, 2006, one month and seven anxiety-filled days after I first asked Neil to escort me to a New York City swing club, I checked into Manhattan's Algonquin Hotel, went up to my room, threw my bags on the floor, grabbed the phone book, flipped open the yellow pages, and searched for sex stores.

Chapter 37

• • • • •

"Where to?" the cabbie asks.

I pull off my eyeglasses, read my list, push my glasses back on—they are my protective wall between the outside and myself—and say, "Twentieth Street between Sixth and Seventh."

I spot Purple Passion when I see its purple décor. Though I hesitate at the door, I urge myself inside. Until an hour earlier, I'd never been into a sex store. Never. Ever. My hour earlier "first" had been small and hotter than hell and had intimidated the hell out of me. Its walls had been the color of the Sunday school rooms of my youth. So had its size and temperature. Then there were its shelves of artfully detailed vibrators. Not my Sunday school room's. The sex store's. Vibrating kangaroos. Vibrating hummingbirds. Vibrating fish. Vibrating lizards. Vibrating swans. A Noah's ark of vibrators. I stared at a rabbit vibrator, its front paws held as in prayer. I flew out the door, raced for the elevator, going the wrong way first, backtracked past the store, down the elevator, onto the street and hailed a cab.

Now, just inside the front door of Purple Passion, a BDSM store, I pause, stunned, wanting to run again. I try to focus on the checkout counter, which is to my left, so that I don't look at the rack of whips to my right. Onward, I tell myself, but what my brain hears is the old hymn "Onward Christian Soldiers." I force myself past racks of leather clothing and into the rear of the store, where there are curtained dressing rooms, their drapes not dropping all the way to the floor. I meander back through the clothing, occasionally glancing up at the wall displays—strips of black leather harnesses for men, hoods, and masks. A kind, heavyset woman approaches me. I inhale and say, "I'm looking for something to wear to a swing club tonight."

She doesn't flinch. Instead, she shows me miniscule black leather skirts and miniscule black leather dresses. *Oh, Lord.* My face contorts as I say, "Uh, I don't have the greatest legs in the world."

She insists that the quality of my legs doesn't matter—everyone will be wearing short skirts. Everyone. Short and fat women. Big and tall women.

I don't care how other women are dressed; I care about how I'm dressed. I run my fingers up and down some rubber dresses. To my astonishment, I love the way they feel. Keeping skin on rubber, I look at their three-figure price tags. "Holy cow! That's out of my budget. I need something cheap." Only God knows if I'll ever wear this stuff again.

I pick through a rack of black leather bras as the saleswoman sorts through the sale dresses. After she shows me a dress or two, I, too, begin flipping through the sale dresses, and then I walk into one of those curtained dressing rooms, drop my Levi's on the floor, and try to slip on a dress. I can't even get it up me. *You must have to be a size two to wear any of this stuff.* I hand the dress to the saleswoman.

She isn't surprised. She knew it wasn't going to fit. It's a medium. But there isn't one large size dress that I like—one that's tailored, classic, like a business suit a reporter would wear on the job. I keep asking myself, *What would Diane Sawyer wear while covering a night at a swing club?* But I know that any network anchor would send her producer to do the sex club research and then show up, dressed in appropriate business attire, do the stand-up, and be on her way. But I also remember Diane Sawyer doing an interview in Europe while wearing thigh-high black leather boots, the very boots that had enthralled Al and his BDSM buddies. I thought the boots had looked ridiculous on her—at least considering that she was wearing them while in reporter mode—and I never saw her in them again. Still . . . she'd worn them.

I return to the rack of black leather bras—their prices closer to my budget. I grab a bra or two and once again go behind the too short drapes, drop my clothes to the floor and try on the bras. "Uh," I mutter through the curtain, "are these things supposed to show the nipples?" I feel I can hear the saleswoman chuckle. The drape opens, and I stand before her with one nipple covered and the other not quite. She tries to politely explain that no, the bra isn't meant to cover the nipples, and that complete coverage isn't the point. *It is to me, though.*

I close the curtain and put my clothes back on as I hear her saying hello to a couple entering the store. I return to the rack of leather bras and thumb through them, while leaning my body backward so that I can watch the interaction between the saleswoman and the couple. The female shucks off her clothes and unabashedly tries on tight, sexy fetish outfit after tight, sexy fetish outfit, modeling them for her male companion, the saleswoman, and whomever happens to be watching—me, the woman holding a black leather demi-bra that doesn't quite cover her nipples.

I find myself standing at the rack of floggers, stroking them. *Whoa*, I say to myself as I realize what I'm doing. But I can't stop running my fingers the length of the leather, then rubber, especially the rubber. I stroke the floggers like I'm petting a horse, again and again and again. And it calms me the same way petting a horse does. I'm so wanting to buy one of those floggers, but the prices!

Many of them are well over $100. Besides, what am I going to do with a flogger, rubber or leather? Hang it from my computer screen along with my old press badges?

I keep stroking as I stare at a rubber mask. I find myself kind of fancying it. To me, it's a Batman mask—it has pointed ears. What girl from the 1960s doesn't have a thing for Batman? *Suzy! What's happening to you?*

I clutch that black leather bra in my hand and stride over to the checkout counter. "I'll take this," I say, still staring up at the rubber garments on display. "I fear I'm developing a rubber fetish."

The salesclerk, a gay young man, laughs. I don't. I pay my $62 bill, sign up for the Purple Passion mailing list, and walk out the door, wondering what in the hell I've just done.

• • • • •

"Went to a BDSM store," I type to Lola. "Have a new black leather bra that, alas, reveals the nipples."

I think about the email that she sent me before I left for New York. "Be careful at the swinger's club. Observe only! Maybe flirt . . . but . . . nothing more."

I think about another email she'd sent me just days before that— she was starting to date again after going through a divorce. "It's amazing," she said, "what some loving attention and affection will do for your self-esteem." And that's when it hits me—Lola had wanted me to get into therapy to learn how to do relationships because she couldn't do without them. I feel a bit betrayed by her. But I also feel maybe I'm not so sick after all.

"So now I'm about to put on my black leather bra," I type, "and I'm going swinging." And I hit "send."

• • • • •

I push my breasts into my leather bra, making sure that they're crammed in enough and the bra cup pulled up enough that my nipples don't show. I cover them with a crinkled velvet blazer, pull on a mid-calf-length skirt—the first skirt I've worn in God knows how many years—and zip up my black knee-high boots. I'm not sure the tops of my four-year-old boots have ever seen the light of day—or in this case the dark of night—since they're usually covered by blue jeans.

I take the elevator down to the lobby of the Algonquin and wait for Neil. Not until two days before I'd left for New York, and after I'd asked Neil to resend me his photograph, did he email me the proverbial close-up photo of his penis, followed by the note: "You can now find me ok even if you happen to be looking down, right? ;-) Don't read anything into my email. . . ."

I didn't. Prior to that, he'd assured me, "I'm planning on being a tour guide, not a player. Please know that I will be looking out for you. You won't get into any trouble."

But ever the true crime writer, now sex writer, I'd given friends the names, addresses, phone numbers, and photographs of Neil, Phoebe, and Phil, in case I went missing. I hadn't, however, given them Neil's penis shot.

I fidget as I wait for him. And wait. And fidget more. When he finally walks through the door, I recognize him immediately. And not because of his penis. His kind face and dark wavy hair look just like his photos. Only two things are different. He has a faint scar on the left side of his forehead, and he's a bit chubbier than in his pictures. "I'm not Fabio. I'm not Flabbio," he'd said in our first phone conversation. "But you can take me out and introduce me around. If I was walking down the street, no one would guess I'm into threesomes."

He was right. With his best dark suit, tie, and overcoat and my blazer, mid-calf skirt, and trench coat, we look dressed for after work cocktails. Immediately I kick into work mode—calm, confident. We step out the door of the Algonquin, into the unusually warm January air, and walk east toward Grand Central Station and the bar he frequents there.

. . . . .

At nine-thirty on Friday night, a few drunken men fall over the bar's counter. Quickly, we order a couple of slices of pizza and begin to chat. Unlike his phone persona, which was stilted, with me practically tugging and begging for information, in person Neil's talkative, forthcoming, insightful, and revealing. Though we touch on the serious—his brother died just two years before in a car accident—mostly Neil keeps me laughing. I giggle as he tells me that at swing parties, Viagra is passed around like M&M's. In my mind, I see the little green and red M&M's guys with their Mickey Mouse–like legs and shoes being passed from the palm of one hairy naked man to another.

Neil interrupts my laughter as he says, "I would never do this if I were married. I don't care what anyone tells you, if they're swinging, there's something wrong in their marriage." An hour later, he grabs his overcoat and a brown paper sack of screw-top wine. Together, we exit Grand Central Station and hail a cab. Reluctantly, Neil gives the driver the address. Reluctantly because Neil worries that his Manhattan coworkers might find out about his swing life. But in the name of research, he's willing to sacrifice in order to introduce me to one of New York's most notorious on-premise swing clubs.

Chapter 38

. . . . .

Piles of garbage line the sidewalk to our right. Three lengths of velvet rope stretch along the sidewalk to our left. Maybe a dozen young, fit, well-dressed men and women stand behind the rope trying to get into the club. *Thank God.* I'm relieved that we'll be among a good-looking crowd and I won't have to be exposed to sagging bellies and pebbled bottoms. Then the yellow taxi stops on the right side of 27th Street. I glance up to see an 1880s-style pub sign hanging from an old building. Discreetly it discloses LeTrapeze. *Oh, man,* I groan. We aren't going to the velvet rope club. We're going to the one that has garbage in front of it.

Neil and I maneuver our way around enough stoves and mattresses to furnish several apartments. "I hope I don't see a rodent," I say, eyeing the trash, fearing it will move. I'm terrified of rodents. In fact, I'm more afraid of a seeing a rat scurry out from under a dirty mattress than I am of seeing a bunch of naked people have sex on a dirty mattress. Still, as we step closer to LeTrapeze, my confidence wanes a bit. Just a bit. I stand a protected few steps behind Neil as he pulls on the building's double metal doors. They're locked. He hits a buzzer and the locks click open. We enter an empty hallway, scuffed and dimly lit. A lone window is on our left. Behind the window, a black man with what looks like a Bluetooth phone attached to his ear tells me, "one hundred and twenty dollars." That's the cost of the $30 membership fee—LeTrapeze is a members only club—plus the Friday night cover charge of $90.

I know from the club's website that we could have brought along an extra woman for an additional $30. But we could not have brought an extra man. Single men are forbidden, and single women aren't allowed unless accompanied by a male/female couple. Neil's my "ticket" to get in. Besides, I would have been too chicken to go by myself. I hear in my head the voice of Angela.

You need to keep your wits about you.

I'm trying to make sure I do, professionally noting everything. The man behind the window asks me no questions, I jot in my head.

"Do you take credit cards?" I ask him.

He acts peeved. "No."

But I need my cash for taxies. And even though I know my next question is stupid, I ask it anyway. "Can I get a receipt?"

His reaction indicates that not only is it stupid, it's ludicrous. But I need that receipt for my taxes. This isn't a sex pleasure trip. It's a tax-deductible sex business trip. I fork over $120 in cash and receive a "temporary" membership card in return. I hope the IRS will accept that as a receipt, despite the fact that my name isn't recorded on it or anywhere else.

In fact, the only thing on the front of the card is a silver and black sticker plugging the club's twenty-fifth anniversary and a stamped expiration date—ninety days after date of purchase. On the back of the card are a few rules, some of which aren't enforced—couples only (obviously not enforced since single women are allowed), no drugs or alcohol permitted (obviously not enforced as Neil carries his screw-top wine), no prostitution, no cameras or recording devices, members must abide by New York State health regulations, and "membership is subject to approval and review" (and we obviously weren't reviewed, unless one counts an irritated glare when asking for a receipt).

A second door buzzes open and Neil and I officially enter LeTrapeze or, as its Internet site stated, the traditional Shakespearean Madison Pub, which has been restored to "turn of the century charm" with stained glass windows, brick walls, wood beam ceilings, and "amenities consistent with modern private clubs."

Blackness and stale cigarette smoke permeate stagnant air. A few steps forward and a left turn past the entryway, there are tiny round tables with brown tops and wobbly chairs painted black. The sparse furnishings look like they were abandoned by an evicted tenant . . . or perhaps picked up from the sidewalk out front. The "landmark" Prince George Hotel, which houses LeTrapeze, had been a welfare hotel in the 1980s, just when LeTrapeze opened. The nonprofit Common Ground still used it to house the formerly homeless.

I wonder if I've done too much pre-research.

The place looks empty. Finally, I spot a couple sitting at one of the tables, trying to look relaxed, enticing, and available. She appears to be over fifty and wears a dark-colored towel around her waist, revealing breasts that sag toward her navel. She smiles at Neil.

Again, I hear Angela in my head. *When three or more people are together sexually, there is so much stimulation that it feeds off itself. That arousal combined with alcohol can result in people tossing out all rules and manners.*

I'd made sure to drink Diet Coke with my pizza, and I'm not about to drink any of Neil's screw-top wine.

I look at the woman's companion. He, too, is of AARP status and is dressed the same as she, his towel looping beneath a medicine ball belly.

A single female needs to watch her back.

Mentally, I tuck my hands behind my butt.

I glance away and over to a TV that hangs from the ceiling. It's showing pornographic movies that no one seems to watch. I turn my attention to a diminutive buffet that lines a portion of a wall—bread, cold cuts, hot mashed potatoes and gravy. "Please cover lower torso at food bar," reads a tacked up sign. I laugh and gag, fearing pubic hair in the mashed potatoes as they're at groin level and there's no sneeze guard. At least some of the food is partially protected by plastic wrap.

Neil and I walk over to a corner bar where club patrons stow their liquor. His screw-top wine, necessitated by the lack of a corkscrew, soon rests in a gray plastic tray of ice next to a bottle of Veuve Cliquot champagne. Paper cups for liquor, soft drinks, and fruit juices and white foam cups for coffee sit atop the bar. I grab a cup meant for the coffee and start to press it against a juice dispenser. Another black man with another Bluetooth-like earphone magically appears and corrects my coffee cup crime.

Wagon wheel chandeliers that look like they were tossed out of a run-down steakhouse barely light the room. The ceiling appears to be hammered tin, its former elegance painted over in black. A glass-enclosed display case stores souvenir LeTrapeze T-shirts. I want to peer into the case and see what's there. But I don't. I don't want to look like a scared novice staring at T-shirts because she's too chicken to look at the people.

I scan to my right, where there's a small dance floor. A few crystals and a disco ball hang over it. The LeTrapeze ball doesn't turn, nor is it lit, as if it burned out and no one cared. A couple of leather-looking couches are positioned to one side. Tired dance music filters through loudspeakers. Just past the dance floor is an empty room with a long, bar-height table surrounded by bar chairs. Several LeTrapeze notepads and pencils are on top of the table, while a nearby TV plays porn that, again, no one watches.

Neil directs me to a back corridor, which leads to the street clothes *not* optional section of LeTrapeze. An elderly white man, his chest covered by a sleeveless undershirt, worn and baggy, a towel hiding his privates, meanders aimlessly as if he's wandering the hallways of a nursing home. A hard-bodied, young, naked black man strolls by, his stride purposeful, confident, and justifiably cocky.

I study the mattresses that carpet the floor of a room with mirrored walls. Outlines of stains mark dark blue sheets. Two couples lie separately having sex. In a similar room there's similar activity, their actions seeming as mundane as strangers chatting in a bus line.

Neil and I walk into the co-ed locker room, where another black man wearing yet another earphone opens a bottom locker and hands us two towels—one a washed out gray-color, the other a faded dark blue, both bath-sized. Duffel bags stuffed with more towels as well as sheets sit on the top lockers. The bags nearly touch the ceiling. I stare at them, wondering how many towels and sheets the club goes through every weekend and how much the club's laundry bill totals, as Neil strips off his suit. I step into the women's restroom. I can breathe in there. Unlike the rest of LeTrapeze, it's clean and light. An open bottle of Listerine capped with a paper sipping cup sits on the counter. I reach for another sipping cup, pour in a swig— wondering if it's safe, leery that it's contaminated with something I don't want. I slug it back anyway, swish for a millisecond, still worried whether or not it's germfree, spit, and reach for the door, while staring at the poster of a gorgeous, well-built, young man that's tacked to the back of the door.

I concentrate on trying to help Neil neatly fold his suit into the tiny half locker, rather than look at his naked, white body.

"Bet this gets really boring," I say to the attendant.

"Yes, it does." He seems to have a photographic memory for which locker he's assigned to which patron. And only he—who has worked long hours into the wee mornings for seven years at LeTrapeze (I ask him)—has the key. After all, where's a naked swinger going to keep a key?

"Do you have a safety pin?" I say.

He pulls open a drawer, and I find a pin. As fast as possible—and

I'm hoping it's Superman fast—I shuck my jacket and skirt, wrap the towel around me, and cram my clothes in the locker. Neil and I walk out of the locker room, past two sex rooms, past a sign that says high heels aren't allowed because they damage the mattresses, past a fourth black man with an earpiece, and begin winding our way up a narrow iron stairwell. Heat and humidity rise with us. The stairwell's packed with people. The upstairs hallway is short and cramped. Men and women, bare elbow to bare elbow, peer into small, doorless rooms.

In each of four rooms there's at least one couple having sex—fellatio in some, intercourse in others, not a condom in sight, not even a tossed wrapper. Toweled voyeurs stop, Neil and I included, watch, and move on like dutiful tourists at a natural history museum—glance at a diorama from a polite distance, move on to the next, glance, move on. Few bother to even pause at two cubicles, each filled with a red sex chair, each unused, each looking as though it has never been mounted, despite the fact that the chairs are built to ease access to the body's orifices.

But everyone halts, seemingly stuck in their steps, where three rooms join in a corner. I don't know if everyone stopped simply because they're at the end of the line, or if they're captivated by the view of the heavy-hipped white woman going down on the well-endowed black man. What stopped me, though, was a putrid smell emanating from the rooms. It hangs there like a mildewed drop cloth. The song lyric "I smell sex and candy" pops into my head, but this isn't an endorphin scent of peppermint and chocolate. It's the odor of old sex in a flophouse.

Despite a few low moans, the sex is blasé—joyless, passionless, even boring, with no close-ups of private parts like the sweating, groaning action of the porno movies playing downstairs.

Neil and I return to the first floor, where the voyeurs clog the bottom of the stairwell as they stare into the mat room. It's a large room carpeted in wall-to-wall mattresses. One of the Bluetooth men tries to urge people on. Neil and I step onto the mattresses.

They sink under my weight like quicksand. We rock and balance our way across the room, every few feet passing silent nude couples in mid intercourse, sit down on the stained sheet covering what feels like foam mattresses, and lean back against the wall, Neil's towel draping open just enough.

"I hope crabs don't jump on me," he jokes.

At least I pray he's jesting.

Eighteen bodies are in the room. Most appear to be in their forties and fifties, most are out of shape.

Then there's the beautiful foursome—a tall, very fit man with thinning gray hair who appears to be in his late fifties or early sixties; his slim, blond, naked female companion who's maybe five to ten years younger than he; her thirty-something, perfectly-tanned-all-over mirror image; and a similarly young, handsome, metrosexual Asian companion with a pierced ear.

The two women kiss, embrace, fondle, caress, and suck each other, their actions exaggerated by the warped mirrors on the ceiling, the cheap reflections distorting their images.

In reality, the older woman's belly protrudes only ever so slightly, a slip of skin barely bags from her upper arms, her breasts droop minutely. The younger woman, not a hair out of place, not a curve that isn't smooth, tenderly kisses the older blonde's shoulders. The older man seems uninvolved. The Asian man unenthusiastically strokes his still-jelling member. A bucket for used condoms hangs on the wall behind them.

A couple to my right, snuggled together, their eyes closed, look like they're napping. Another couple finishes their sex and strikes up a conversation with the couple next to them, the freshly excited woman sitting up and jabbering as though she's at her neighborhood coffee klatch.

But I can't stop watching the beautiful foursome. The flawless blond women continue entwining and licking each other's perfection, revealing the tattoo on the younger woman's lower back. She mounts the Asian man, keeping her back to him, her face to the woman.

Her jeweled belly chain flashes with each bounce as she humps the man and kisses the other woman.

I glance at the crowd gathered by the stairwell. A very few of the white couples wear robes. Not one black man is unattractive or out of shape. Many of the toweled white men are hairy or plump and balding. The sagging older woman who'd expressed interest in Neil gazes toward him as she reaches beneath her husband's bulbous stomach, pushes aside his towel, and touches his limp penis. I can't look.

I turn back to the beautiful foursome. The young blonde now faces her Asian man. The older blonde rides him with her, their torsos pressed back to breasts, their rhythms in perfect synchronization.

"I'm thirsty," Neil says, as he moves to his feet.

"I'll go with you."

"No, that's okay."

But moments later, he stands at the edge of the mattresses, signaling me. Couples have to enter and exit together, the LeTrapeze rules state.

"I'll go and you can stay," purrs the woman who's interested in Neil as I squeeze by her.

Neil jokes that I should "take one for the team." I smile and ignore his comment just as I did the woman's.

He and I move into the empty room near the dance floor. While I sit at the long, Formica-topped table, scribbling tiny notes to myself on a tiny piece of paper, Neil bums a cigarette and lighter from a fully-clothed woman. She sits unattended in an easy chair next to the dance floor. When Neil leaves to pour himself a paper cup of his screw-top wine, the woman's companion arrives and approaches me wanting back his cigarette lighter.

We talk briefly. He's attended many lifestyle events, he says.

"I want to learn everything there is about the lifestyle."

"As a single or a couple?" he asks.

I shrug my shoulders. "Either."

Emotionally, he steps back. "This isn't really a swingers' club," he says.

"Then what is it?"

He glances at the pencil in my hand and the tiny piece of paper that I try to cover with my palm. "I'm not being interviewed here, am I?"

Again, I shrug. "Maybe."

"That's the last thing I want." He picks up his lighter and walks away.

Neil and I make one last tour through the sex rooms. Upstairs, a man has his briefs lowered just enough to have intercourse, his hips and tightie whities rising in the air. On the way back downstairs, stuck in the crunched crowd staring into the mat room, I hear a woman's voice. "Oops, I dropped my towel"—I glance at her face—"on purpose." She looks me in the eyes. I edge by her.

As the attendant opens our locker, the striking young blonde stands near us, pulling on her blue jeans.

"The Asian man you were with—" Neil says.

"You mean *my husband*," she tersely retorts.

Neil tries to back up. "I thought I knew him from work."

"He has his own business." There's disdain in her voice.

"How often do you come here?" I ask.

"About every other week." She softens a bit, revealing a model smile with straight white teeth. Her blond hair is expensively cut.

"Why aren't you at Checkmate?"

She looks at me, a hard question mark on her face.

Checkmate is another Manhattan swing club that I'd heard about. It promotes itself as the club of choice for the beautiful people. "Well, you're obviously a very attractive couple." It claims to have a rope line that allows in only the young, gorgeous, toned, trendy, well-dressed, and prestigious. "I hear it's difficult to get into." I figure that's why Neil and I are at LeTrapeze rather than Checkmate. Well, that and the fact that he's been to LeTrapeze before—with the wife of the foreign diplomat Phoebe told me about.

The diplomat liked Neil to bring his wife to the club, have sex, observe every detail, then return home and report all the orgasmic facts.

I wonder if he'd like to see my tiny scribbled notes.

"We just call ahead and tell them to put our names on the list," the perfect young blonde says, before her husband walks in and our conversation abruptly ends.

The attendant points to a dark-haired man I'd noticed throughout the night. He walked around the lounge area, a towel wrapped around his waist, lingered in the first-floor hallway but never near the sex rooms, in and out of the lounge, in and out of the lounge, and always by himself. I couldn't figure out why. He was silver screen handsome and one of the few white men there who was well built and had a look of class. In fact, that's the reason I'd kept looking at him. "He's washed his hair and taken five showers," the attendant says.

I laugh and notice a couple staring at me, the man rubbing his hands.

On the way out, Neil and I stop by the bar to pick up his screwtop wine. As we do, the woman with the sagging breasts approaches him. In a skirt and blouse with glimmering beaded earrings dangling from her ears, she's much more attractive. Narrow, rectangular black glasses surround her eyes.

Neil comments that they're sexy.

"That's what people tell me. I started to put in my contacts but decided I'd go secretarial sexy instead."

She notes that her glasses are similar to my small red eyeglasses and wants to know what I'd been wearing beneath my towel.

"I'm sorry we never got together," Neil says to her.

"Me, too. Maybe next time." She smiles nicely.

He asks for her number.

She laughs as she glances over at her husband, he, too, looking better now that he's covered in a suit and tie. But seconds later, they leave.

Perhaps it was my black leather, knee-high boots that I refused to take off, even in the sex rooms that didn't allow high heels . . . or the way my towel was securely attached to my black leather demi-bra by my borrowed safety pin . . . or my cotton Jockey underwear that I wore beneath my towel, but I'd just spent three hours in a swing club and not one person made a move on me.

· · · · ·

I sat in Grand Central Station the next afternoon wondering if I was ever going to figure out the swinging signals. I'd noticed the dazzling backside of the young blond woman when she first walked through the lounge. She was the only shapely and tanned woman in the place wearing a beaded gold thong. But I wondered how she and her husband had gone from one trot through the lounge area to immediately having sex with the only other beautiful couple there. Was that one essentially nude walk-through enough to set up the perfect pairing? Had there been a hand signal? A touch to the shoulder? A caress of the hip? A sentence, a phrase, a word exchanged? Or had they made plans to meet there?

I pondered on what Rose had taught me—the women are supposed to do the talking, so approach the woman, not the man. Maybe that's why the blonde had been more open to me rather than Neil. Maybe that's why the woman with the sagging breasts had asked me what I'd had on underneath my towel. Perhaps my own emotions had been stifled and that's why I couldn't figure it all out. I grabbed my baggage and boarded a train for Connecticut. I had Phoebe's DNA party to attend.

Chapter 39

• • • • •

The hotel in Connecticut is a typical nondescript, roadside business
hotel—neat at first glance, stained carpets and stained furniture on
second look, but free breakfast and free Internet service. I know
that because I sit in my room studying its every detail, doing anything I can to keep from going downstairs to the bar. I plug in my
computer. I hook it up to the free Internet. At 8:06 P.M., I send Lola
an email. "I didn't even flirt last night. And no one flirted with me.
How humiliating. . . . In fact, the swing club was rather boring."

Just a few hours before, I stood on the Brewster North train
platform, shivering in the cold winter's night, waiting for Phoebe and
Phil. As I waited, my brain obsessed over the events of the past few
months, and my trust in Phil and Phoebe began to ebb. Probably,
more accurately, my trust in Phoebe. I thought about how she was
searching for that elusive unicorn. *Uh-oh. Don't think about that.*

I paced. I reminded myself that Phoebe was an attentive mother
who shuttled her daughters to cheerleader practice. I reminded
myself that she was a New York Giants fan, just like any typical
New Yorker. I remembered that she had a male porn star friend she
could call anytime to "scratch that itch." *Don't think about that*

one either. I forced myself to picture her snow-covered home. She'd sent me a photograph of it. It looked so normal—white, frame, colonial. I thought about how she'd written a letter to a radio station asking for Christmas help for an Iraq War veteran. *Now, that's good. Keep thinking on that one.* I remembered the Christmas package she'd sent to Phil in Iraq—wine, porn, and mistletoe. "Maybe he can get lucky," she'd said.

I thought about an email I'd sent her after I'd reread their swinger profiles. "How does one do double vaginal penetration?"

She'd laughed. "It is actually very easy and it feels fantastic, the added girth really hits the sensitive inner walls and sends me off.

"You can sit on a cock facing the guy and have the 2nd guy enter from behind. You can do the reverse cowgirl sitting on the bottom guy with your back against his chest and be facing the top guy as he enters.

"Shit, you can lie on your side and get a sandwich made of yourself or you can have both guys suspend you up in the air as you are impaled on them."

A little blue car zoomed into the night, its headlights flashing on me. Phil jumped out, grabbed my bags, and we were off—Phoebe at the wheel, Phil beside her, and me in the backseat.

We stopped for a quick steak dinner, with Phoebe inhaling her red meat between loud words explaining our upcoming night—one woman just had surgery, is on painkillers, and having her period, but she'd be there for oral. We'd all meet in the bar around eight-thirty to loosen up. The bartender at the hotel was swing friendly and sometimes joined the party. Phoebe got away for the weekend by telling her kids she was working. We needed to hurry. We had to run by the liquor store for some Shiraz wine and tequila. My head whirled like a carnival teacup. Did I even eat?

We zipped to the store, with Phil behind the wheel. *Thank God.* He was a much safer driver.

When we checked into our hotel rooms, Phoebe was disappointed that suite 223 had been reserved for them, not their usual DNA room of 314. She promised me they'd make 223 into a new DNA room. As we departed to our separate rooms on separate floors, she reminded me to meet them in the bar at 8:30 P.M. to loosen up. I didn't want to loosen up. I wanted every single one of my wits about me.

. . . . .

I step into the shower and stand there, hot water spraying over my body as I shampoo and shave every hair that the average Southern Baptist thinks of shampooing and shaving . . . and think about Phoebe's words: "Our bag of toys does not include a weed whacker." That makes me laugh and feel like I'm wearing a chastity belt. But I still don't want to go down to that bar.

The phone rings. It's Phil and Phoebe wondering where I am. I mutter some excuse and eventually, slowly, lay a pair of red silk pajamas on the bed. Despite Phoebe's silky robe suggestion, I'd brought pajamas because I don't want anything accidentally flying open. I put on my panties. I put on my bra. I put on my button-fly Levi's blue jeans. I pull on my black boots and zip them up tight to my knees. I put on and button up my pajama top. It's big and boxy so that it covers my torso as seductively as a large, brown paper sack. And as for my pajama bottoms, years before, to make them more comfortable to sleep in, I got my mother to cut them off at the knees and hem them. Now, whenever I wear them, they hang down my thighs like a pair of baggy basketball shorts. I roll them up as if I'm packing them for an overseas trip. I place my tape recorder on top of them, and carefully wrap the bottoms around the recorder. Well after nine o'clock, the planned start time of the actual suite party, I finally exit my hotel room.

I take the elevator down one flight and wander the hotel corridors until I find room 223. I stare at the numbers. I roll up the sleeves of my pajama top. One roll. Two rolls. Three rolls. I inhale, force my right arm up, curl my hand into a loose fist, and urge it to knock.

I wait. No one answers. I press my ear to the door. Silence.

Reluctantly I go down to the bar. It's crowded and noisy, no place for a tape recorder to catch anything intelligible. Worse, there's no place to hide my pajama bottoms. I barely step into the room, so that I can dangle one arm out the door and hold my shorts behind the door frame.

The bartender—a heavy-set woman, not their usual swing-friendly guy—calmly shuttles drinks between locals and Phoebe's guests. The drinkers are so mingled that I can't tell which are locals and which are members of Phoebe's party, especially since she loudly jokes with all and invites everyone within shouting distance to join us upstairs.

"What room number?" ask a couple, their elbows on the bar, their eyes carefully watching Phoebe.

"Two twenty-three," she says.

I turn my focus on Becky, the only person I know for sure is with Phoebe's group. She's a dark-haired, casually dressed, divorced mother who showed up just to meet me. As she slowly sips a beer and Phoebe knocks back a cocktail, I turn on my recorder, hoping I'll get *something* on the tape other than Phoebe's alcohol-laced voice. Becky works full-time, attends graduate school part-time for her MBA, and swings with a married man. *Only* with him, absolutely *never* without him, she emphasizes, so she will not be going up to the suite. They have a relationship that's more than just sex, she insists.

Phoebe, not so softly, whispers into my ear several times that Becky's relationship with the married man is just sex but Becky can't accept that reality.

Becky protests.

I think about Phoebe's relationship with Phil and how they don't let any of their swinger friends know that Phil's married.

Becky repeatedly tells me she's lonely and wants to find Mr. Right. She also tells me many times that she's upset I don't swing.

"Why don't you?"

I watch the couple that Phoebe spontaneously invited to the party mere moments ago. They pay their tab, creep out the front door, and into their car, driving away in the cold dark. I turn back to Becky and give her my same old spiel—if I did, it'd ruin the book; either I'd write that swinging is the best thing since sliced bread or that swinging destroyed my life; I'd lose all objectivity and credibility.

Like everyone else, Becky doesn't buy my explanation.

By then, Phoebe's ready to move the party upstairs.

"I'm going to stay down here and talk to Becky some more," I say, postponing the inevitable as long as I can. "I'll be up in a little while."

. . . . .

Finally I return to the door of suite 223. I clutch my tape recorder, carefully rewrapped in my red silk pajama bottoms, in my left hand and extend my right hand toward the door. But it won't go there. Again, I find it rolling up my pajama sleeve. One roll. Two rolls. Three rolls. As it does, I keep thinking about how Phoebe had said that she gets everyone naked as soon as they walk through the door. I look at my watch. Eleven P.M. I spent two hours with Becky. I *know* that by now everyone in that room *is* naked. I don't want to get naked. I don't even want to change out of my Levi's—my safe, sex interview, work clothes—into an embarrassing pair of "basketball shorts" in the bathroom of a hotel suite that's filled with naked people. I wonder if I could roll up the shorts, like I had my sleeves, just a bit so that they don't look so stupid. But then people would see my sushi white, cellulite thighs. *Hell*. I don't understand why this is so much scarier, so much more intimidating, than the swing club. I want Neil, my protector. *Do it*, I order my hand. It knocks on the door. The door swings open.

Chapter 40

· · · · ·

Raucous laughter pours out as I step into the room. I nervously scan the suite full of swingers. The room's brightly lighted. I can clearly see that everyone's fully clothed. I take a step forward and stand next to Phoebe.

She motions to a young, heavyset woman who wears blue jeans and a conservative striped sweater. "This is Mary."

"I'm lit," Mary laughs as she leans toward me like she's about to fall out of her chair. She has shining, Hispanic eyes and an even brighter smile.

Phoebe proceeds with the introductions as I numbly stand there and scan the room for an empty seat. The only one is on the couch, next to a woman whose dyed beaver brown hair is permed into tight curls. They look like if I smashed them against her head they'd spring back into place, like a natural sponge.

"Tricia," Phoebe says to introduce the woman. I don't want to sit next to Tricia. She wears red, thigh-high stockings and has "tube sock tits" that aren't lifted one iota by her red halter minidress. At least that's the way Phoebe describes the breasts when we're alone. Phoebe has never forgotten or forgiven that Tricia "cock-blocked" her at a previous swing party, meaning she prevented Phoebe from having sex with men Phoebe wanted. I plop down in the doorway, next to Phoebe and Phil. Only Phoebe notices as I unfold my pajama bottoms just enough to click on my tape recorder, shove it and my basketball jammies under a table, and turn to blue-jeaned Mary.

"The movie *Harry Potter*," Mary roars as she describes her first date with her boyfriend David, a cute, tubby, thirty-year-old Native American from Oklahoma who sits next to her. "I love Harry Potter," she yells. Her pierced tongue glints in the light when she laughs. "Kids all over the goddamned place so you can't like cop a feel of the cock there—"

"Without breaking some sort of law," shouts Griff, an average Joe.

"Ask Pee-Wee Herman," Phoebe throws in.

"So we're doing the whole like coming really close to kissing but not quite—"

"Mommy, where's her hand?" Griff hoots, mimicking a child in the theater. "There's no popcorn in his lap."

"So we go to Outback Steakhouse, and we're just about to go in for dinner, and I lean in and I'm like, 'Can I just kiss you on the cheek?' And he grabs me by like the back of my hair." She acts it out. "We're making out in the Outback parking lot for a good half hour. Then we go in for dinner and we're all like—" She indicates that they're all over each other. "Yeah, over dinner and then back out in the Outback parking lot making out for another good half hour.

"Then we go—where'd we go?" She turns to David. Clearly he's crazy about Mary, who keeps her hand tucked between his legs, frequently rubs his penis, and overshadows him at least for this night. But David doesn't seem to mind one bit.

"Starbucks," she says, "right? Making out outside of the car at Starbucks. Apparently he got a thumbs-up from like a ten-year-old." Delight erupts. "We go to the bar, making out outside the bar. We actually have a crowd of people outside the Jeep."

"Were they cheering?"

"Were they cheering?" she asks David.

"Only the ten-year-olds," someone cracks.

"They were watchin', I'll tell you that," she continues. "He goes to drop me off at home. . . . He's outside of the Jeep on his knees in the gravel—before knee surgery mind you—chowing down like a man about to be executed, his last meal. . . . And then he gives me the chaste kiss good night. Yeah, after all of that! . . . And we've been together ever since. It's been love ever since. And he gave me a compliment: 'What a good little cocksucker you are.' I think it's a compliment," she cracks.

Mary's chair is pushed against a large table that I practically sit under in utter silence. I know part of me is quiet because I'm in reporter mode, trying to be unseen so that I don't become a part of the story, while trying to listen and observe and take in every detail. But I think another part of me is in shocked silence. I'm not sure I've ever met anyone like Mary.

My gaze moves from her to a clear acrylic dildo swirled with blue that sits on top of the table, side by side the array of sodas, liquor, and snacks. I reach up, curl my fingers around the dildo as though it were an exhibit to be examined, and pull it down to me.

"It's hers," Phoebe says. "Mary brought that."

I place it back, feeling as though I've touched something that Mary doesn't want me to touch.

"It's just pretty," Mary practically moans, "and it feels soooooo good. Oh, my god."

She then laughs about her time working in a porn shop, and everyone jumps in, hooting riotously, as conversation loudly pinballs from dildos to porn movies, from bestiality to anal sex.

"Oral sex is sex and so is anal," Phoebe shouts.

Talk then moves to children—almost everyone in the room has children, ranging in age from one to eighteen—and teaching their children about sex and condoms.

Mary grabs the stage again as she regales the group with the grilling she took from David's ten-year-old daughter over where Mary slept, now that she's living with David.

When Griff's wife Emily remarks to Mary, "You're a lot of fun," Mary rejoins, "And we're not even naked yet."

In fact, everyone's still fully clothed. I lean over to Phoebe. "When are things going to get going?"

"Hey, this is way too much fun," she says with a dismissive wave of her hand. Phoebe looks so different from the photograph she emailed me months before. For that matter, so does Phil. His photo didn't reveal one bit about his personality, which is that of a sweet and methodical Southern gentleman.

Even better, the man I watch is a tall, gorgeous Southern gentleman wearing black slacks over long legs and a tight-fitting black sweater that hugs a hard body. His goatee is perfectly trimmed. And his hair doesn't look buzz cut, just closely cropped.

Although Phoebe looks younger than she did in her photograph, this night she appears worn and heavy, with disheveled blond strands—and not disheveled in a sexy way. She seems rumpled in slacks and a white blouse, its buttons left open to reveal her large breasts.

"I want porn star tits," Mary suddenly announces.

From that, Phoebe starts talking about penile implants and Viagra, specifically recounting an emergency room story from the hospital where she works. "And this guy was recreationally using Viagra."

I think about Neil's Viagra/M&M's story.

"And it was up and it was not coming down," Phoebe continues. "And his girlfriend had taken his clothes. So he not only had a hard-on in twenty-degree weather, but he was naked in the car. They had to come out with a gown for him!"

Everyone howls until Phoebe thinks she hears someone outside the door. The room goes silent, like children afraid they're going to get caught. But then they just use the lull as an excuse to go outside and smoke.

With only a handful of people in the suite, Tricia looks into my face and invites me to sit next to her. Hesitantly, I do. But swiftly I learn that she's been to many lifestyle conventions and clubs including LeTrapeze. In fact, she proudly insinuates that she's tried everything. She claims she's forty-eight. She looks closer to fifty-eight, which Phoebe says she is. And Tricia's irritated that things haven't gotten going sexually at this party.

"Are you into men or women?" she asks.

I falter, thinking about the man at LeTrapeze who backed away when I gave him a wishy-washy answer. I fear if I say men, I'll turn Tricia off and she won't talk to me anymore. And if I say women, I fear she'll think I'm interested in her. I'm not. I don't know what to say. But before I have a chance to come up with anything, Tricia demands, "Well, you'd better decide," and immediately scoots away from me and closer to her boyfriend Ray, who keeps his arm around her.

Ray's a nice-looking black man, six feet, four inches tall, with a slight belly from fifty-two years of life. His mustache is flecked with a bit of gray. His face is sweet and kind.

I look at the people in the room and ask Tricia, "Who interests you?"

"I find that who you talk to and who you have sex with have no relation at all," she says as if shoving closed a window and snapping it locked.

"Well, does anyone interest you?" I persist.

I look at Emily. I'd barely noticed her before, since Mary had captured everyone's attention and Tricia had commandeered mine. Emily's a forty-one-year-old mother wearing a tight-fitting black top that zips up the front, a black box-pleated miniskirt, black fishnet stockings, and black booties with sharp, pointy toes.

I feel self-conscious in my shapeless pajama top.

Dark red lipstick heavily accentuates a charismatic smile and straight, white teeth. Long, brunette hair is layered into waves. At least her hair looks brown. When Phoebe refers to Emily as a brunette, Emily quickly corrects her and says she's a redhead.

Emily usually stands next to Rita, who I'd also barely noticed. More honestly, perhaps I hadn't noticed these two women because they're the best looking females in the room and they seem like popular types. Girls who were popular in high school sometimes intimidate me.

My popular teen theory is reinforced by the fact that the two are inseparable. I think they're best friends who, like cheerleaders, planned their nearly matching attire. But they just met tonight, and Rita's long hair is closer to black and isn't layered like Emily's. Her shoes are high heels rather than booties, and her fishnets are a larger mesh.

"Now, *those* are fishnets," Griff remarks, not as an insult to his wife, but more as an off-the-cuff comment implying "We should buy those for you next time."

And finally there's Lex. He's tall, thin, and nondescript and spends his time standing near a table covered with beer bottles and bragging about multimillion-dollar beach homes, Ferraris, and big fancy swing parties he and his wife Rita have thrown. I'm told he's a psychiatrist. I don't believe it. He doesn't seem to have the IQ for medical school or the demeanor of an MD. And he has a constant Beavis and Butthead marijuana laugh—"huh, huh, huh, huh." I have a hard time putting him together with Rita, a sultry California girl who loves horses. Plus, Lex has gray teeth and constantly smokes, stinking up the non-smoking room we're in despite the fact that Phoebe has asked him not to. Frequently, though, he leaves the room to smoke, usually with Rita, Emily, and Griff.

Still, Tricia refuses to answer me. So as she pouts on the couch and ESPN plays on the TV, Ray and I talk about sports. He's a high school football coach at the very school where he was a football star.

Filtering through the air are Emily's words that this is her first swing party.

"Are you serious? This is your lose your virginity party? Good God!" Phoebe cries out.

She and Emily proceed to gripe about the cliquish private swing parties they've heard about where one has to apply and be approved—frequently on the basis of looks—and about swingers who refuse to kiss on the mouth.

"What's up with that?" Phoebe pointedly says, knowing that Rita and Lex's swapper profile states in all capital letters that they don't kiss on the mouth.

"You're sucking somebody's dick," Emily throws in. "You can't kiss somebody on the mouth!"

"What's with this bullshit about kissing on the mouth being too personal? What's more personal than penetration? It's okay to stick it in my ass, but don't kiss me on the mouth."

Phil confesses that he made a no kissing on the mouth note by Lex and Rita's names.

"You take notes?" Phoebe laughs.

Phil not only takes notes, he frequently gets up and tidies the room. I like this man. He's classy, especially when compared to Lex, whose "huh, huh, huh" is growing more exaggerated and beginning to sound like Woody Woodpecker. By now, conversation seems like it's never going to end, and it's becoming irrelevant, boring white noise. Thank God for Ray.

Softly he speaks about his fondness for bondage and domination. His voice is so calm that being flogged doesn't sound frightening at all.

David moves Mary into the bathroom. Their noises signal sex. When they return to the living room, she laughs, "I don't drink well."

Ray seems oblivious to them, as he continues his domination conversation. "For example, somebody's who's a single parent, who has to work, who has to make all the decisions, all the responsibilities, they're in charge of everything, they can't wait to have all that stuff relieved and have someone else be in charge."

"Do y'all ever practice it together?" I glance toward Tricia.

"Not D and s. She's not into submission . . . but she likes to have her pussy lips clothespinned closed."

"Really?" My voice is calm, but my right hand desperately wants to move to shield my groin.

"Yeah, I've had seventeen clothespins on her."

I don't want to visualize that. *Not at all.*

Thank God I'm distracted by David as he pushes Mary across the room, almost like she's a wheelbarrow. He apologizes that she's had too much to drink. She was nervous about the party, he explains. Mary scoops up her acrylic dildo, and David scoots her out the door, everyone but Tricia lamenting that the life of the party has left.

"She was blotto," Phoebe announces when Emily, Rita, Griff, and Lex return from smoking once again. Each time, they're gone longer and longer. We surmise they're hooking up in Emily and Griff's room . . . until I sit down next to Griff.

Griff's a nice farm boy from Iowa—polite, easy to talk to, and easy to smile, revealing teeth that are almost as perfect as his wife's. His closely shaved hair and goatee are dusted gray, despite the fact that he's only forty years old. He works for a telecommunications firm.

Like Tricia, Griff wonders when the action is going to start. He says he tried to get things going by unzipping his wife's top, but she slapped his hand. And they tried to maneuver into sex with Rita and Lex on their various smoking trips, including a trip to their room. But nothing worked. So here he is sitting next to me, frustrated, and it's 1 A.M.

I, too, am frustrated. All I can think about is all the time and money I've spent to travel to Connecticut and for what—nothing but a bunch of strangers sitting around talking. I have to do something. I turn to Griff. Already, I've confessed to him my real reason for being here—to research and write a book about sex in America. "I've got an idea," I say. "Strip poker."

But there are no playing cards. I wander into the bedroom, where a second TV is tuned to ESPN. In here, the lighting is low, a lavender candle burns, and condoms lie on the nightstand on each side of the king-sized bed—splayed out like an assortment of mints.

I guiltily scoop up all the condoms and take them back to the living room.

I say guiltily because I'm about to do what no ethical reporter should ever do—I'm about to manipulate the news to get my story.

Griff finds a pen and I try to mark on the outer edge of one foil wrapper. The ink disappears into the foil like water into a Sprite. I tear one corner slightly, grab an empty six-pack container, toss in the condoms, and shake them up. Condoms fall from the folds of the six-pack. Griff picks them up and dumps them into a plastic bag. I pass them around, making sure everyone but me picks one, and announce, "Whoever has the torn condom—"

"Has to jump in the hot tub naked," Griff finishes.

Big ole Ray gets the torn condom. He begins pulling off his shirt, and the next thing I know, I'm standing in the bathroom and he's in the bathtub. His body fills it so that suds slosh everywhere and there's barely room for a now nude Phoebe. I can't watch. I know Phoebe too well. I step out of the bathroom as she plops into the water beside him. I walk back into the living room, turn around, and see Ray fully clothed. "Why are you dressed?"

"Because everyone else is."

Again, I turn around. This time I see Tricia wearing a conservative brown coat over her red halter dress. Still frowning, she's obviously ready to leave. Seconds later, Tricia and Ray are out the door—her cock-block against Phoebe successful once more.

I sit back down next to Griff. "What's plan B?" I ask.

Across from us, Emily and Rita sit side by side, smiling, staring at us, giggling, staring at me, whispering, staring at me, laughing.

"What?" I say.

The light in Emily's eyes flickers. Her grin teases. It's as though she's chopping up fine lines of cocaine and wordlessly taunting me, tantalizing me to come take one little taste. Not forcing me, not begging me, not ordering me, not ridiculing me, but simply coaxing with the gleaming flirtation of a drug I've never tried.

I cross my legs, exposing the soles of my boots.

Emily rises from her chair, walks over to Griff and me, and brushes by us, grabbing, then releasing the foot of my boot. Moments later, she stands over my still-booted foot with my toes between her legs, centimeters from her crotch. Rita moves close to watch. They both laugh and smile, temptingly. Neither moves away.

I reach for the zipper of Emily's top and slowly pull it down.

Chapter 41

· · · · ·

All I'd wanted to do was get the party going and get my story. Then I'd fly back home to Texas, sit alone in my little town house, and type up my notes. Nothing in my life would have changed except that I would have watched some strangers have sex, laughed, and gotten out of true crime. Nothing. Other than the fact that I'd breached my journalistic ethics by manipulating the story. But I'd deal with that later.

As I unzipped Emily's top, she grinned and murmured something I couldn't decipher through everyone's light whoops and hollers. They were thrilled and relieved that something was finally happening. She stood there and bored her twinkling eyes into mine. Life began to move in a slow-motion blur. Someway, somehow, sometime, Emily's top came off. I reached behind her and fumbled with the snaps of her black bra. I got one hook undone. Griff tried to do the rest, but she stopped him, wanting me to do it. I tried again. I *may* have unfastened one more, but my fingers fumbled. Griff finished for me.

Emily signaled Rita to come closer. They quietly slipped to their knees and kissed on the floor. Air and sound ceased.

Griff and I watched as the women were at my feet.

Rita's top came off.

I looked up. Everyone had inched close to the two women, encir-
cling them, watching them, contented grins on all their faces. Even
huh-huh-huh Lex was hushed, as he stood behind his wife, smiling.
This was what I wanted. Action. With me not involved.

But Emily moved back to me. Did she kiss me? Unbutton my top?

I'm not sure. I hadn't had a thing to drink other than water, so
I can't blame my memory—or what happened—on alcohol.

"You are so sexy," Emily whispered in my ear. No one had ever
called me sexy. "You are so beautiful." No one had ever called me
beautiful.

Her words were my alcohol.

You need to keep your wits about you.

She tried to place her breast in my mouth. I didn't want it. I
wouldn't let her.

"Will you let Griff fuck you? He has a really nice penis."

I didn't want that either. But I did. But I didn't. I didn't answer
her. What was Rita doing? Maybe Rita tried to participate. Emily
moved back and forth between us. At some point, Emily tried to
unbutton my jeans. Did she and Griff unbutton them together? I
know I flailed and pushed people off and away from me. Was I
laughing while I did it? Like I had with the man who'd pulled out
his penis and said, "Do you have a place where I can stick this?"

Years later, he'd told me my laughter had said yes, though my
words had said no. Was my laughter saying yes? Or was I silently
saying yes?

Someone unbuttoned my jeans, but Emily, thank God, couldn't
get them off of me. My boots were in the way. She, Griff, and Phoebe,
unzipped, pulled, and tugged off my boots. They then lifted me into
the air, yanked, and off came my jeans.

*The reality is scary, though, because you become dehumanized.
Emotions are put on the back burner.*

My memory gets even more confused from there. I know I stood up many times—at least three, maybe four, maybe five times—buttoned my top, grabbed my jeans, put them back on, buttoned them, and then they stripped off my clothes again. I know Phoebe laughed and smiled every time. I know Emily kept whispering, "You are so sexy. You are so beautiful." I drank her words. "Will you let Griff fuck you? He has a really nice penis. He knows what to do with it."

Yes. No. Yes. No. Aloud, I said nothing.

Phoebe and Phil spread a blanket on the floor. They kept trying to get people to move to it so as not to get knee burn. No one moved. So Phoebe tried to get everyone into the bedroom. Somehow, everyone began to ease in there. I stood. As I walked to the bedroom, dazed, I heard Griff tell Lex I was writing a book.

"Yeah, right," Lex said, unbelieving.

I was ticked.

· · · · ·

And from there, I'm confused about what to tell you. What to admit.

The truth shall set you free.

But not that kind of truth.

I think about my family and how they'll be hurt by this story. I think about my career and how it will be damaged by my truth.

There are differing standards of conduct for male and female journalists.

I think about my Christianity and how others will question the legitimacy of my faith.

Rose, am I a hypocritical Christian?

Yes, I answer myself. And I'm not laughing.

· · · · ·

It's now more than five years since I was at that swing party in Connecticut. It seems like several lifetimes ago. Rose is no longer a part of my life. She got married and became—as far as I know—happily monogamous. Perhaps my jealousy killed our friendship.

Perhaps my Christianity did. Perhaps it was neither. Maybe it was just me. The only truth I know is that I still love her and I miss her desperately.

Lola is barely a part of my life. I haven't seen her in God knows how many years. On very rare occasion we exchange a brief email. But we never discuss anything of import. And we never, ever discuss sex. I miss our old friendship.

As for my shrink, well, here's what happened . . .

*   *   *   *   *

The mood can change quickly. It can be dead as a doornail for one and a half hours, and then sex is happening.

When I walked into that darkened bedroom, I don't think I had the intention of having sex. But I'm not sure. I *think* my intention was to simply lie there and watch, take as many mental notes as possible, then run back to my room and write them up. But my memory differs a bit from the notes I typed and scribbled that night and over the next few days.

My memory says I said no, no, no, and my no's were ignored.

My notes say I was naked, feeling defeated, thinking why the hell not have sex, I've gone this far. And then there was the fact that someone desired me. That was more than dewdrops for a parched soul. But my notes say it wasn't so much that I gave in to desire, it was more that I gave up.

I flopped down on the bed, crossways, toward the foot of the bed, Emily next to me, on my right. I rolled my head to the left. Phoebe, in a lightweight wrap robe, sat on the edge of the bed giving Phil, who was naked, a blowjob. I had no idea that they'd shed their clothes. He was beautifully built from head to toe and definitely in between. Definitely in between. I felt I was gawking. I rolled my head back to my right. Emily was on top of me. Rita lay next to her.

Emily forced one of her breasts into my mouth. I didn't know what to do with it. It was large, soft, flattened and molded against my nose and mouth as though a breast form had been filled with peanut butter and smashed into my face—a peanut butter breast pie. I couldn't breathe. I tried to move my head away.

"You're so wet."

I didn't want to be wet. But I wanted to be wet. I wanted to be able to feel.

That side of me seems to have died.

I looked back at Phil and Phoebe. Rita sucked him, briefly, before Phoebe took over again. Every so often I heard him tell Phoebe she was sucking him perfectly. Some time, some way, Griff and Lex had stripped off their clothes. Lex's body was long, too skinny, sickly white and tattooed.

"Will you let Griff fuck you?" Emily continued whispering. "Will you let Griff fuck you?" I felt her putting my hand on her. I pulled away because all my fingers felt was a hard mound covered in razor stubble. It felt weird—the hardness. I was soft there.

"Will you let me lick you?" she whispered. "Just one little lick."

Eventually, I barely uttered yes.

A single female needs to watch her back.

"Don't let the Beavis and Butthead guy touch me," I kept whispering.

She promised she wouldn't.

"Will you let Griff fuck you?" Emily asked me again and again.

I couldn't say yes. It was wrong.

I barely nodded yes.

It's okay to sublimate on occasion, but use caution and common sense.

"Make sure he wears a condom."

She said they never party without one.

I closed my eyes, trying to feel the moment. I couldn't. I opened them and saw Phoebe and Phil sitting there, watching us.

Every so often Emily moaned with pleasure. I didn't know what was being done to her. It seemed like Lex might have been entering her. I was disgusted that she'd let him do her. Maybe Lex was messing with his wife, too. And all this time I was thinking Emily only wanted me because I was a challenge, constantly trying to stop things, constantly trying to get away.

Then Griff couldn't enter me. He didn't seem upset. He just got some lube. Then he got more lube, so much that I felt like I was at the gynecologist, and said so. Everyone laughed and said it's not supposed to be like that, it's supposed to feel good and fun. I joked that maybe I have a really great gyno.

Finally, Griff entered me. It hurt like burning hell. I told Emily that it hurt. She got him to pull out. He eventually tried again. I tried to bear the pain. It was excruciating. I couldn't take any more. I put my hands together to call time. Everyone pulled back. I got up, found my clothes, as a robed Phoebe and a naked Phil followed me around, Phoebe helping me find my underwear.

"How are you?" she said.

I briefly looked at her. She was smiling. I wasn't. I turned away. "Disappointed with myself."

· · · · ·

At 3 A.M., I flipped on my laptop, took a bath to try to scrub myself clean, and sat down at the keyboard. "I fucked up," I emailed Lola.

That fast, ten years of celibacy down the drain—washed away faster than I could scrub my bathtub.

"Big time," I typed.

Flushed. Gone. Forever. I couldn't have it back.

But then . . . with just a little bit of flirtation . . . oh, God, it felt so good to be flirted with. It had been so long. Oh, God.

"My body, soul, and spirit are feeling it." I hit "send."

And as for my career, I'd just blown that. Not only had I manipulated the news by getting the party started, I'd crossed the professional and ethical lines of getting involved with the story *and* getting involved with my sources.

I crawled into bed to see if I could bury myself in sleep.

· · · · ·

The next morning, Phil took me to the train station. We barely mentioned the night before. Instead, we talked about Iraq. By the time I got back to the city, I was about to drop with exhaustion. The dark circles I had under my eyes from LeTrapeze were now plum-colored. I wanted to hide in bed.

But Phoebe emailed me that afternoon. "Sooooo," she asked, "what was your take on the evening? We had an absolute freaking blast. GREAT group."

I sat in silence, staring at her words.

Late that night, I phoned Lola. She didn't answer. I left a message. But I couldn't wait that long to talk. I typed, "I need to talk to a CHRISTIAN friend. The only other friend who I can talk to about this is a bi, poly atheist and isn't who I really need to listen to right now. She's like, yippee, when I'm like whoa . . . yea! . . . oh, you really fucked up in a bunch of ways . . . but you learned something important . . ."

I kept the something important to myself.

Lola responded within six minutes. "Sounds like you got in over your head? I'm sure you have done nothing that will permanently cause you harm. And you know if you decide you made some bad decisions God forgives EVERYTHING."

I read that last line over and over. I tried to phone Lola again and only got her answering machine. "God forgives EVERY-THING." I read those words for twelve minutes, until I finished my email reply to her and hit "send." "I succumbed and did what you told me not to do. . . . My shrink is going to have a field day on Thursday. I try not to think about it. Scared I'll cry."

I tried to distract myself with chitchat. "This hotel has a

FABULOUS apple tart. Wish I could get one and a glass of milk. Alas, the kitchen is closed."

I closed my email: "I've been trying to remind myself for nearly 20 hours that God forgives. But family doesn't. The two-sided Suzy must continue. Integration? What's that?"

* * * * *

The next day, Phoebe emailed me again, wanting to know how I was doing, begging to know what I'd thought of the party, and asking me to think about joining her and Phil in Las Vegas.

I plainly wrote her, "I'm still NOT planning on playing. More convinced of that than ever." I emailed Lola, "Still nearly start to break into tears every so often. . . ."

I coped with alcohol, music, and food. By myself, I went to Birdland, had a martini, and listened to jazz. Then I went to The Palm and ate a steak and drank a glass of wine. I walked back to my hotel. I thought about how nice it was to have someone tell me that I'm sexy and beautiful. I thought about the Old Testament proverb that said pride goeth before a fall. My ego had definitely triggered a fall. I took a bath, and ordered up an apple tart and a glass of nonfat milk.

And I anxiously awaited my Thursday shrink appointment.

But it didn't happen. My shrink called and canceled. I had another week to think, fret, and cope on my own. I emailed Lola. I downed a burger and fries. I tried to write, but though I hadn't felt at the time that LeTrapeze and the swing party were surreal, I was beginning to realize they were, especially the party. I couldn't remember details. I could remember seeing a small penis and love handles, but I couldn't remember when everyone's clothes had come off. I could remember seeing a female body that looked like it had lost a lot of weight, with loose belly skin. But . . . "Is that accurate?" I asked Phoebe. I couldn't even remember what her body looked like, though I did remember Phil's. Most of all, I wanted to know what made someone decide to have sex with another. There seemed to be no need for physical attraction, just a vacant hole. . . .

I emailed Lola, "I regret what I did Saturday for the sake of the book and my journalistic integrity." I regretted what it would do to my family and my relationship with them. "But otherwise, I don't regret it at all (as long as I don't come down with a life-changing STD).

"I learned some big time things about me. For one, sex—even with mountains of lube—is horrifically, physically painful for me. As almost always, it felt like a dagger that was just below molten temperature. God, it hurts so badly."

Lola comforted me, telling me I should only do what I felt good doing, not what I thought I should do, or what others would do, "or what someone told you God would say. Your heart and your soul are what you have to live with." Sex, she said, was not bad or sinful or evil. "The problem with it is that usually there are complicated feelings involved with it. And people get hurt. If you are enjoying it, and feeling loved and respected, then I'm not sure it's 'bad' for a 50-year-old woman to enjoy sex."

But she warned me, too. "Everyone wants to be wanted and desired. It heals the soul. Just don't sell your soul for something phony and ultimately hurtful to you long term. The most important thing I can say to you is respect yourself. No matter what you decide is the right thing for you to do."

And I waited for my shrink appointment.

*　*　*　*　*

Finally, it happened. . . .

Afterward, I raced to Jack-in-the-Box for a grilled sourdough burger and curly fries. Yes, the appointment had been that bad. My shrink's body had jerked when I told her about my night in Connecticut. She'd then denied that she'd reacted. And in truth, she hadn't physically reacted at the mention of Griff. Her body had jerked only when I said Emily, too. And I don't know why, but I feel compelled to add that Griff and Emily did me. I didn't do them. And *only* Griff and Emily. Does that absolve me of any sin? Absolutely not.

The following week's appointment was even worse. I sat down in my usual spot. There was a putrid smell there. To get away from the odor, I moved to the other end of the couch, which placed me closer to my shrink. She said that was me being seductive—that I was attracted to her. I wasn't. I felt she was trying to force transference that didn't exist.

She complained that I didn't jump back into the sex talk of the previous week. I couldn't. I had work to do, and dealing with all of that confusion, and confusing feelings, destroyed my ability to think. I knew I'd fucked up. I knew I'd gotten too involved in my research. I at least wanted some credit for recognizing that.

I talked about the acne that covered my face. My shrink thought I was making small talk. No! I was talking about my innermost being, all my ugliness that's on display, and no matter how hard I try, it won't go away.

I left enraged.

Rose encouraged me to drop my shrink. I felt I needed to stay in therapy. I had too much to work on. I still hated touch. I still couldn't do relationships. And I was still trying to be the person my family wanted rather than the one God intended. So I returned to celibacy, kept going to therapy, and kept working on the book, despite the fact that my shrink repeatedly told me I was living in fantasyland if I thought it would ever succeed. Ironically, she told me I should write a memoir. I don't think she meant a sex memoir.

Five months after Connecticut, I fired her. I knew I had more research to do. I knew it would once again tempt my secret desires. And I presumed I would give in to the temptation. I didn't want—or need—to pay someone to berate me for that. I emailed Lola, "Think I'm headed for a period of serious self-destruction and a nervous breakdown. Think I'll get a Prodigal Son welcome home?"

But the Prodigal Son had to repent. And I was no longer repentant.

Maybe that's when Lola and I started losing contact. Or maybe it was because she got married again.

All I know is that five years later, my hands tremble as I try to write this ending. I stand. I pace. I weep. I pray. I sit down. I try again. And I do it all over. I *know* that Jesus will love me no matter what. And He *knows* how much I've prayed over this book, particularly the ending—especially how much to reveal about that night in Connecticut.

I told all because my soul knows that what you do in the dark comes out in the light. In truth, there are no secrets.

But what makes the tears fill my eyes and my voice quaver is my family. My mother—that strong, godly woman—did have kidney cancer, and she survived. At eighty-six years old, she's still cooking, cleaning, and nurturing.

And as I sit here at my desk, staring at my computer screen, part of me wonders if the writing of this book is my teenaged rebellion again. This time forty years too late. I also wonder if it's a way to sever ties with my mother so that when she dies it won't hurt so much. Yes, I know, thinking—hoping—that it won't hurt so much *is* fantasyland.

But the truth I learned about me that night in Connecticut is something I can no longer keep secret. And that truth is that I'm not dead inside.

I'm not dead inside!

Acknowledgments

If I thanked everyone who helped create this book, my thank-yous would extend for another three hundred pages. Through email, by phone, and in person, I communicated with hundreds of people throughout the United States, meeting many, as you know, via the Internet. But what you don't know is that I also met Americans from all walks of life at swing and kink conventions and events in New Jersey, Nevada, Florida, California, Mexico, and Jamaica, and more than twelve hundred people, from every state in the union, answered my online sex survey, which you can still access through my website, www.suzyspencer.com.

It's been a wild, fun, sometimes excruciating, and definitely life-altering eight-year ride filled with laughter, tears, and new friendships that I cherish. Though I have some regrets, and many embarrassments, I'm not sure I would change any of it. And for this fabulous trip, I must thank Nicholas Ellison, my literary agent. As you know, this book was Nick's idea.

Nick, truly, I thank you. My memory is not short when it comes to those who help me. I will *always* be grateful to you.

Denise Silvestro, my beautiful editor who acquired this book for Berkley Books, has believed in it—and me—when seemingly no one else has, including me. Denise eased, then "forced," this book from a journalistic overview of sex in America to a memoir, something that this journalist fought every single day and every single sentence. Denise's patience, encouragement, and toughness have been boundless as she coached me through countless rewrites, stretching my abilities as a writer, and urging me to reveal more of myself. I love Denise's humor. I love her empathy. I love her acceptance of me both as a writer and human being.

Denise, words of gratitude fail me. "Undying" is all I can think of when I think of you. I hope you understand what I'm trying to say.

I also want to thank Berkley editorial director Susan Allison, whose patience is surely equal to Denise's. Thank you, Susan, for allowing this book to germinate in my soul and become a manuscript worthy of publication. I know—Denise has made it very clear—that this book would not have happened without you. Thank you.

I also know that this manuscript would not be nearly the book that it is without the strong editorial hand of Meredith Giordan. Denise whacked tens of thousands of words from the original manuscript. And when Denise's and my eyes were crossing and our brains were too muddled to edit one more word, Meredith came to our rescue, cutting thousands more words and doing it with such finesse and insight that she definitely made this a much better and more cohesive book. I shout to everyone in New York City: MEREDITH GIORDAN IS A GREAT EDITOR AND DESERVES A PROMOTION.

Thank you, too, to the Berkley publicity team of Craig Burke, vice president and director of publicity; Julia Fleischaker, director of publicity; and Heidi Richter, senior publicist. Never before have I had a publicity team. Y'all are a dynamite dream. And to Heidi, in particular, thank you for listening to all of my ideas and putting up with my too many emails.

I also need and want to thank my personal support team. Novelist Carol Dawson declared this a memoir before Denise even did. In fact, before Denise even heard about the book. So for eight years Carol has been with me as a dear friend and believer. In fact, the opening of the book is Carol's idea. Thank you, Carol. Thank you. I could not do without you.

"Lola," "Rose," the "Jazz Cowboy," Vanessa Leggett, and God knows how many other people I've left out, were all there for me in the early stages of the book. Thank you all.

In the final stages, Elizabeth Brinton and Myra Morris Jackson were my rocks of emotional support. Liz, Myra, thank you! My Facebook